MW01253439

ANTI-INFLAMMATORY DIET

FOR BEGINNERS

The 2 Week Meal Plan to Naturally Restore
the Immune System and Heal Inflammation
with 300 Proven Easy Recipes

Sebastian Carlus Murphy

Table of Contents

Introduction

The anti-inflammatory diet is not just for weight loss, although you may lose weight while on this diet. It is not a limited, three-week trek to push current inflammation from the body. It is not a false, quick leap to health. It provides a specific, new approach to your life: a way of life complete with all the nutrients and minerals, calories, and proteins that one needs to live well and happily. The anti-inflammatory diet components will help boost your overall health by providing the necessary nutrients and inflammation-fighting compounds to allow your body to heal itself and maintain proper balance. You will begin to notice changes in how you look and feel. You will have a sense of renewed energy. Your skin will take on an unmistakable healthy glow. Your body will be working correctly, producing new healthy cells, and calming the chaos of inflammation within your system. To follow the anti-inflammatory diet and reap the health benefits, you must understand yourself.

Symptoms of Inflammation

The main signs of inflammation include; heat, redness, pain, swelling, and muscle-function loss. These symptoms depend on the inflamed body part and its cause. Some of the widespread signs of chronic inflammation are:

- Frequent infections
- Weight gain.
- Body pain.
- Insomnia
- Fatigue
- Mood disorders like anxiety and depression
- Gastrointestinal problems like diarrhea, constipation, and acid reflux disease.

The typical symptoms of inflammation rely on various inflammatory effect problems. When the body defends mechanism which influences the skin, it causes rashes. When you are dealing with arthritis rheumatoid, it affects the joints. Most of the signs and symptoms experienced are fatigue, tingling, joint pains, stiffness, and swelling.

Similarly, when experiencing inflammatory bowel, it typically influences the digestive system. Its usual signs consist of bleeding ulcers, anemia, weight loss, bloating, pains, diarrhea, and stomach pains. With multiple sclerosis, the condition occurs on the myelin sheath, which covers the nerve cells. Its signs consist of problems when passing out stool, double vision, blurred eyesight, fatigue, and cognitive issues.

If you encounter any of the symptoms and the health problems, you could be suffering from inflammation. Many people link it to joint pains like arthritis, which can be signaled by swelling and aches. The problem is related to health problems, not just swollen joints. Nevertheless, all soreness is not bad. For instance, acute inflammation is vital throughout recovery from a twisted and puffy ankle.

It is easy to detect Chronic inflammation signs and causes. Insomnia, genetic predisposition, your food intake, and other individual habits can cause it. Similarly, inflammation resulting from allergic may also develop in your gut.

Below are some of the possibilities that you may be having it:

- If you always feel tired to the extent of not having enough sleep, not getting enough nap, or sleeping excessively.

- Do you experience time-to-time aches and pains? It may also signify that you have arthritis.

- Are you experiencing any pain in the gut or stomachache? The pain may create inflammation. Gut inflammation may also cause cramping, bloating, and loose stools.

- A swollen lymph node is another sign of inflammation. These nodes lie in the neck, armpits, and groin, which swell if there is a problem in your system. When you have a sore throat, your neck nodes lump because the body's defense system has sensed the condition. These lymph nodes react since the body is fighting the infection. The nodes reshape as you heal.

- Is your nose stuffed up? If indeed, maybe it is a symptom of irritating nasal tooth cavities.

- Sometimes, your epidermis may protrude because of internal inflammation.

Foods to Eat

If you already eat an appropriate healthy diet, you will have no trouble incorporating these foods into your meals. You may already be enjoying them and need a few tweaks to increase their presence in your meal planning. Some of the right foods that prevent and reduce chronic inflammation are as follows:

Omega 3 Fatty Acids

Omega 3 fatty acids are found in fish and fish oil. They calm the white blood cells and help them realize there is no danger to return to dormancy. Wild salmon and other fish are good sources; It is recommended to eat them three times a week. Other foods rich in Omega 3s are flax meal and dry beans such as navy beans, kidney beans, and soybeans. An Omega3 supplement may be helpful if you are not able to ingest enough of these foods.

Fruits and Vegetables

Most fruits and vegetables are anti-inflammatory. They are naturally rich in antioxidants, carotenoids, lycopene, and magnesium. Dark green leafy vegetables and colorful fruits and berries do much to inhibit white blood cell activity.

Protective Oils and Fats

Yes, there are a few oils and fats that are good for chronic inflammation sufferers. They include coconut oil and extra virgin olive oil. Butter or cream is also acceptable to consume. Ghee, made from butter, is even better because it has the lactose and casein removed – the very ingredients cause so much trouble if you have lactose intolerance or wheat sensitivity.

Fiber

Fiber keeps waste moving through the body. Since the vast majority of our immune cells reside in the intestines, it is essential to keep your gut happy. If that doesn't provide enough fiber, feel free to take a fiber supplement.

Miscellaneous

Eat foods with spices and herbs instead of bad fats and unsafe oils. Spices like turmeric, cumin, cloves, ginger, and cinnamon can enhance white blood cells' calming. Herbs like fennel, rosemary, sage, and thyme also reduce inflammation while adding delicious new flavors to your food.

Fermented foods like sauerkraut, buttermilk, yogurt, and kimchi contain helpful bacteria that prevent inflammation.

Healthy snacks would include a limited amount of unsweetened, plain yogurt with fruit mixed in, celery, carrots, pistachios, almonds, walnuts, and other fruits and vegetables.

Foods to Avoid

While many foods should be included in your diet to aid in reducing chronic inflammation, there are also some foods that you must avoid to help keep the inflammation down.

Processed foods and sugars are two of the biggest culprits when it comes to inflammation in the western diet. Processed foods are highly refined, causing them to lose much of their natural fiber and nutrients. They are often high in omega 6, trans fats, and saturated fats, increasing inflammation.

Sugar is one of the worst offenders when it comes to increased inflammation. Not only does it hide in many foods, studies have found that it is also very addictive. Because of this, you should expect to go through a withdrawal phase when you remove it from your diet. It can often cause headaches, cravings, and sluggishness. Give yourself some time to allow your body to work through it. You don't have to remove natural sugars from your diet entirely, but you should work towards eating them a few times a week and at no more than one meal per day.

Most fried foods, especially deep-fried foods, should be avoided as well. Usually, they are cooked in processed oils or lard and are coated in a refined flour that promotes inflammation.

You will want to pay attention to foods known as nightshades. Nightshades can be anti-inflammatory, but some people are sensitive to them; if you find you seem to have more inflammation after consuming nightshade, you may want to begin to make substitutions in your recipes.

Breakfast

Breakfast Pitas

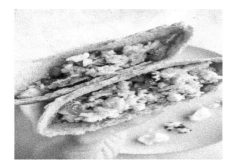

Preparation Time: 4 minutes

Cooking Time: 6 minutes

Servings: 4

Ingredients:

8 egg whites

2 c. bell peppers, chopped (any color)

1 tsp. garlic powder

1 tsp. onion powder

1 c. raw spinach (cook if you prefer)

2 tsp. extra virgin olive oil

4 whole-wheat pita pockets

Directions:

Put the olive oil to a large sauté pan and place over medium heat. When the oil is hot in glistening, toss in the bell pepper and sauté for about 3 minutes or until tender. Add in the spinach now (if you want it cooked) and sauté for about 1 to 3 minutes or just up to the sides starts to wilt.

Place the egg whites into a small bowl, whisk well. Add in spices; whisk well. Pour the egg mixture into the sauté pan and scramble everything together.

Remove from heat and stuff ½ to 1 c. mixture into a pita pocket and serve.

Nutrition:

Calories: 153 kcal

Protein: 12.4 g

Fat: 3.41 g

Carbohydrates: 19.32 g

Almond Scones

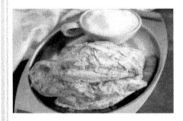

Preparation Time: 10 minutes

Cooking Time: 20 minutes

Servings: 6

Ingredients:

1 cup almonds

1 1/3 cups almond flour

¼ cup arrowroot flour

1 tablespoon coconut flour

1 teaspoon ground turmeric

Salt, to taste

Freshly ground black pepper, to taste

1 egg

¼ cup essential olive oil

3 tablespoons raw honey

1 teaspoon vanilla flavoring

Directions:

In a mixer, put almonds then pulse till chopped roughly

Move the chopped almonds in a big bowl.

Put flours and spices and mix well.

In another bowl, put the remaining ingredients and beat till well combined.

Put the flour mixture into the egg mixture then mix till well combined.

Arrange a plastic wrap over the cutting board.

Place the dough over the cutting board.

Using both of your hands, pat into 1-inch thick circle.

Cut the circle in 6 wedges.

Set the scones onto a cookie sheet in a single layer.

Bake for at least 15-20 minutes.

Nutrition:

Calories: 304

Fat: 3g

Carbohydrates: 22g

Fiber: 6g

Protein: 20g

Oven-Poached Eggs

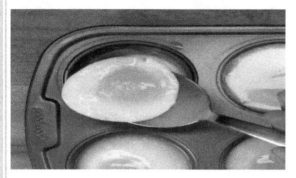

Preparation Time: 2minutes

Cooking Time: 11minutes

Servings: 4

Ingredients:

6 eggs, at room temperature

Water

Ice bath

2 cups water, chilled

2 cups of ice cubes

Directions:

Set the oven to 350°F. Put 2 cups of water into a deep roasting tin, and place it into the lowest rack of the oven.

Place one egg into each cup of cupcake/muffin tins, along with one tablespoon of water.

Carefully place muffin tins into the middle rack of the oven.

Bake eggs for 45 minutes.

12

Turn off the heat immediately. Take off the muffin tins from the oven and set on a cake rack to cool before extracting eggs.

Pour ice bath ingredients into a large heat-resistant bowl.

Bring the eggs into an ice bath to stop the cooking process. After 10 minutes, drain eggs well. Use as needed.

Nutrition:

Calories: 357 kcal

Protein: 17.14 g

Fat: 24.36 g

Carbohydrates: 16.19 g

Cranberry and Raisins Granola

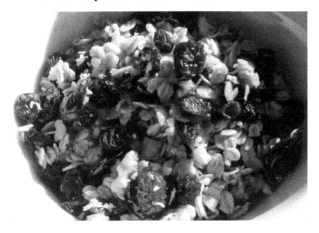

Preparation Time: 15 minutes

Cooking Time: 20 minutes

Servings: 4

Ingredients:

4 cups old-fashioned rolled oats

13

1/4 cup sesame seeds

1 cup dried cranberries

1 cup golden raisins

1/8 teaspoon nutmeg

2 tablespoons olive oil

1/2 cup almonds, slivered

2 tablespoons warm water

1 teaspoon vanilla extract

1 teaspoon cinnamon

1/4 teaspoon of salt

6 tablespoons maple syrup

 1/3 cup of honey

Directions:

In a bowl, mix the sesame seeds, nutmeg, almonds, oats, salt, and cinnamon.

In another bowl, mix the oil, water, vanilla, honey, and syrup. Gradually pour the mixture into the oats mixture. Toss to combine. Spread the mixture into a greased jelly-roll pan. Bake in the oven at 300°F for at least 55 minutes. Stir and break the clumps every 10 minutes.

Once you get it from the oven, stir the cranberries and raisins. Allow cooling. This will last for a week when stored in an airtight container and up to a month when stored in the fridge.

Nutrition:

Calories: 698 kcal

Protein: 21.34 g

Fat: 20.99 g

Carbohydrates: 148.59 g

Leek & Spinach Frittata

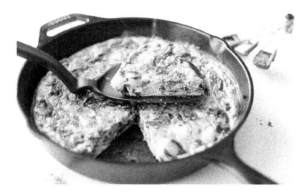

Preparation Time: 10 minutes

Cooking Time: 15 minutes

Servings: 4

Ingredients:

2 Leeks, Chopped Fine

2 Tablespoons Avocado Oil

8 Eggs

½ Teaspoon Garlic Powder

½ Teaspoon Bail, Dried

1 Cup Baby Spinach, Fresh & Packed

1 Cup Cremini Mushrooms, Sliced

Sea Salt & Black Pepper to Taste

Directions:

Set the oven to 400°F then get an ovenproof skillet. Place it over medium-high heat, sautéing your leeks in your avocado oil until soft. It should take roughly five minutes

Get out a bowl, and whisk the eggs with your garlic, basil, and salt. Add them to the skillet with your leeks, cooking for five minutes. You'll need to stir frequently.

Stir in your mushrooms and spinach, seasoning with pepper.

Place the skillet in the oven then bake for 10 minutes. Serve warm.

Nutrition:

Calories: 276

Protein: 19 g

Fat: 17 g

Carbs: 15 g

Cherry Chia Oats

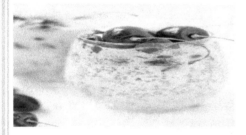

Preparation Time: 10 minutes

Cooking Time: 20 minutes

Servings: 2

Ingredients:

¼ Teaspoon Vanilla Extract, Pure

2 Tablespoons Almond Butter

8 Cherries, Fresh, Pitted & Halved

1 Cup Quick Cook Oats

2 Tablespoons Chia Seeds

¼ Cup Whole Milk Yogurt, Plain

1 ¼ Cup Almond Milk

Directions:

Mix all of together the ingredients until they're combined well.

Seal in two jars and refrigerate for twenty-five minutes before serving.

Nutrition:

Calories: 564

Protein: 22 g

Fat: 32 g

Carbs: 27 g

Banana Pancakes

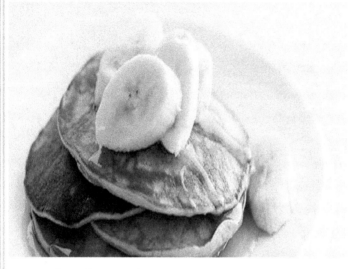

Preparation Time: 5 minutes

Cooking Time: 15 minutes

Servings: 2

Ingredients:

2 Eggs

1 Egg White

1 Banana, Ripe

1 Cup Rolled Oats

2 Teaspoons Ground Cinnamon

1 Tablespoon Coconut Oil, Divided

1 Teaspoon Vanilla Extract, Pure

½ Teaspoon Sea Salt

Directions:

Get out a food processor, grinding your oats until they make a coarse flour.

Add your cinnamon, egg whites, eggs, banana, vanilla, and salt. Blend until it forms a smooth batter, and then heat a small skillet over medium heat. Heat a half a tablespoon of coconut oil, and then pour your batter in. Cook for two minutes per side, and continue until all of your batter has been used.

Nutrition:

Calories: 306

Protein: 15 g

Fat: 15 g

Carbs: 17 g

Baked French Toast Casserole

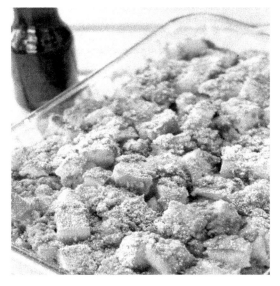

Preparation Time: 20 minutes

Cooking Time: 45 minutes

Servings: 12

Ingredients:

1 lb. French bread

1 cup of egg white liquid

6 eggs

1/3 cup maple syrup

1-1/2 cups of rice milk,

½ lb. raspberries

½ lb. blueberries

1 teaspoon of vanilla extract

¾ cup strawberries

Directions:

Slice the bread into small cubes. Keep them in a greased casserole dish.

Add all the berries. Only leave a few for the topping.

Whisk together the egg whites, eggs, rice milk, and maple syrup in a bowl.

Combine well.

Put the egg mixture on the top of the bread. Press the bread down. All pieces should be soaked well.

Add berries on the top. Fill up the holes, if any.

Refrigerate covered for a couple of hours at least.

Take out the casserole half an hour before baking.

Set your oven to 350 degrees F.

Now, bake your casserole uncovered for 30 minutes.

Bake for another 15 minutes covered with a foil.

Let it rest for 15 minutes.

Serve it warm with maple syrup.

Nutrition:

Calories 200

Carbohydrates 31g

Cholesterol 93mg

Total Fat 4g

Protein 10g

Fiber 2g

Sodium 288mg

Sugar 10g

Salmon Burgers

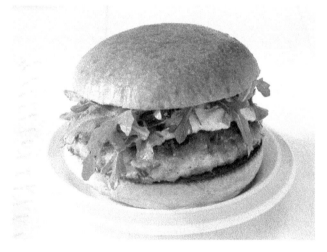

Preparation Time: 15 minutes

Cooking Time: 8 minutes

Servings: 3

Ingredients:

1 (6-oz. can) skinless, boneless salmon, drained

1 celery rib, chopped

½ of a medium onion, chopped

2 large eggs

1 tablespoon plus 1 teaspoon coconut flour

1 tablespoon dried dill, crushed

1 teaspoon lemon

Salt, to taste

Freshly ground black pepper, to taste

3 tablespoons coconut oil

Directions:

In a substantial bowl, add salmon and which has a fork, break it into small pieces.

Add remaining ingredients excluding the for oil and mix till well combined.

Make 6 equal sized small patties from the mixture.

In a substantial skillet, melt coconut oil on medium-high heat.

Cook the patties for around 3-4 minutes per side.

Nutrition:

Calories: 393

Fat: 12g

Carbohydrates: 19g

Fiber: 5g

Protein: 24g

Quinoa & Beans Burgers

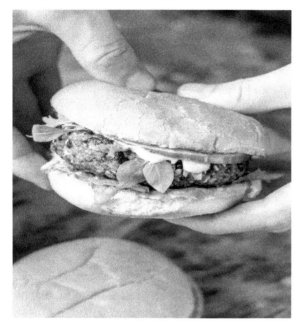

Preparation Time: 15 minutes

Cooking Time: 55 minutes

Servings: 12

Ingredients:

½ cup dry quinoa

1½ cups water

1 cup cooked corn kernels

1 (15 oz.) can black beans, drained

23

1 small boiled potato, peeled

1 small onion, chopped

½ teaspoon fresh ginger, grated finely

1 teaspoon garlic, minced

½ cup fresh cilantro, chopped

1 teaspoon flax meal

1 teaspoon ground cumin

1 teaspoon paprika

1 teaspoon chili flakes

½ teaspoon ground turmeric

Salt, to taste

Freshly ground black pepper, to taste

Directions:

In a pan, add water and quinoa on high heat and provide to a boil.

Lower the heat to medium and simmer for around 15-twenty or so minutes.

Drain excess water.

Set the oven to 375°F. Line a sizable baking sheet that has a parchment paper.

In a sizable bowl, add quinoa and remaining ingredients.

With a fork, mix till well combined.

Make equal-sized patties from the mixture.

Arrange the patties onto the prepared baking sheet in the single layer.

Bake for around 20-25 minutes.

Carefully, alter the side and cook for about 8-10 minutes.

Nutrition:

Calories: 400

Fat: 9g

Carbohydrates: 27g

Fiber: 12g

Protein: 38g

Spicy Marble Eggs

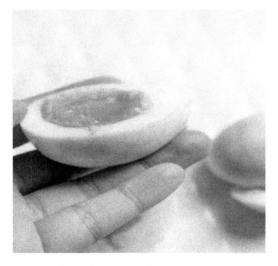

Preparation Time: 15 minutes

Cooking Time: 2 hours

Servings: 12

Ingredients:

6 medium-boiled eggs, unpeeled, cooled

For the Marinade

2 oolong black tea bags

25

3 Tbsp. brown sugar

1 thumb-sized fresh ginger, unpeeled, crushed

3 dried star anise, whole

2 dried bay leaves

3 Tbsp. light soy sauce

4 Tbsp. dark soy sauce

4 cups of water

1 dried cinnamon stick, whole

1 tsp. salt

1 tsp. dried Szechuan peppercorns

Directions:

Using the back of a metal spoon, crack eggshells in places to create a spider web effect. Do not peel. Set aside until needed.

Pour marinade into large Dutch oven set over high heat. Put lid partially on. Bring water to a rolling boil, about 5 minutes. Turn off heat.

Secure lid. Steep ingredients for 10 minutes.

Using a slotted spoon, fish out and discard solids. Cool marinade completely to room proceeding.

Place eggs into an airtight non-reactive container just small enough to snugly fit all these in.

Pour in marinade. Eggs should be completely submerged in liquid. Discard leftover marinade, if any. Line container rim with generous layers of saran wrap. Secure container lid.

Chill eggs for 24 hours before using.

Extract eggs and drain each piece well before using, but keep the rest submerged in the marinade.

Nutrition:

Calories: 75 kcal

Protein: 4.05 g

Fat: 4.36 g

Carbohydrates: 4.83 g

Nutty Oats Pudding

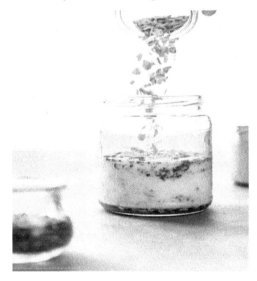

Preparation Time: 5 minutes

Cooking Time: 0 minutes

Servings: 3 -5

Ingredients:

¼ cup rolled oats

1 tablespoon yogurt, fat-free

1 ½ tablespoon natural peanut butter

¼ cup dry milk

1 teaspoon peanuts, finely chopped

½ cup of water

Directions:

Using a microwaveable-safe bowl, put together peanut butter and dry milk. Whisk well. Add in water to achieve a smooth consistency. Add in oats.

Cover bowl with plastic wrap. Create a small hole for the steam to escape.

Place inside the microwave oven for 1 minute on high powder.

Continue heating, this time on medium power for 90 seconds. Let sit for 5 minutes.

To serve, spoon an equal amount of cereals in a bowl top with peanuts and yogurt.

Nutrition:

Calories: 70 kcal

Protein: 4.25 g

Fat: 3.83 g

Carbohydrates: 6.78 g

Gingerbread Oatmeal Breakfast

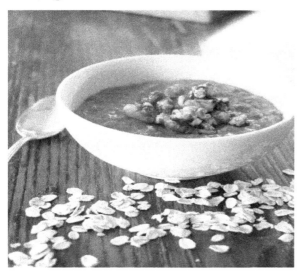

Preparation Time: 10 minutes

Cooking Time: 0 minutes

Servings: 4

Ingredients:

1 cup steel-cut oats

4 cups drinking water

Organic Maple syrup, to taste

1 tsp ground cloves

1 ½ tbsp. ground cinnamon

1/8 tsp nutmeg

¼ tsp ground ginger

¼ tsp ground coriander

¼ tsp ground allspice

¼ tsp ground cardamom

Fresh mixed berries

Directions:

Cook the oats based on the package instructions. When it comes to a boil, reduce heat and simmer.

Stir in all the spices and continue cooking until cooked to desired doneness.

Serve in four serving bowls and drizzle with maple syrup and top with fresh berries.

Enjoy!

Nutrition:

Calories: 87 kcal

Protein: 5.82 g

Fat: 3.26 g

Carbohydrates: 18.22 g

Apple, Ginger, and Rhubarb Muffins

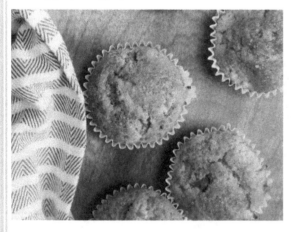

Preparation Time: 15 minutes

Cooking Time: 25 minutes

Servings: 4

Ingredients:

½ cup finely ground almonds

¼ cup brown rice flour

½ cup buckwheat flour

1/8 cup unrefined raw sugar

2 tbsp. arrowroot flour

1 tbsp. linseed meal

2 tbsp. crystallized ginger, finely chopped

½ tsp. ground ginger

½ tsp. ground cinnamon

2 tsp. gluten-free baking powder

A pinch of fine sea salt

1 small apple, peeled and finely diced

1 cup finely chopped rhubarb

1/3 cup almond/ rice milk

1 large egg

¼ cup extra virgin olive oil

1 tsp. pure vanilla extract

Directions:

Set your oven to 350Fgrease an eight-cup muffin tin and line with paper cases.

Combine the almond four, linseed meal, ginger and sugar in a mixing bowl. Sieve this mixture over the other flours, spices and baking powder and use a whisk to combine well.

Stir in the apple and rhubarb in the flour mixture until evenly coated.

In a separate bowl, whisk the milk, vanilla, and egg then pour it into the dry mixture. Stir until just combined – don't overwork the batter as this can yield very tough muffins.

Scoop the mixture into the arrange muffin tin and top with a few slices of rhubarb. Bake for at least 25 minutes, till they start turning golden or when an inserted toothpick emerges clean.

Take off from the oven and let sit for at least 5 minutes before transferring the muffins to a wire rack for further cooling.

Serve warm with a glass of squeezed juice.

Enjoy!

Nutrition:

Calories: 325 kcal

Protein: 6.32 g

Fat: 9.82 g

Carbohydrates: 55.71 g

Anti-Inflammatory Breakfast Frittata

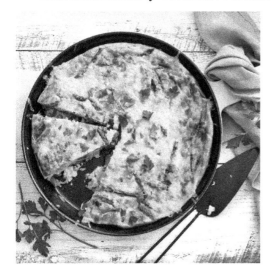

Preparation Time: 10 minutes

Cooking Time: 40 minutes

Servings: 4

Ingredients:

4 large eggs

6 egg whites

450g button mushrooms

450g baby spinach

125g firm tofu

1 onion, chopped

1 tbsp. minced garlic

½ tsp. ground turmeric

½ tsp. cracked black pepper

¼ cup water

Kosher salt to taste

Directions:

Set your oven to 350F.

Sauté the mushrooms in a little bit of extra virgin olive oil in a large non-stick ovenproof pan over medium heat. Add the onions once the mushrooms start turning golden and cook for 3 minutes until the onions become soft.

Stir in the garlic then cook for at least 30 seconds until fragrant before adding the spinach. Pour in water, cover, and cook until the spinach becomes wilted for about 2 minutes.

Take off the lid and continue cooking up to the water evaporates. Now, combine the eggs, egg whites, tofu, pepper, turmeric, and salt in a bowl. When all the liquid has evaporated, pour in the egg mixture, let cook for about 2 minutes until the edges start setting, then transfer to the oven and bake for about 25 minutes or until cooked.

Take off from the oven then let sit for at least 5 minutes before cutting it into quarters and serving.

Enjoy!

Baby spinach and mushrooms boost the nutrient profile of the eggs to provide you with amazing anti-inflammatory benefits.

Nutrition:

Calories: 521 kcal

Protein: 29.13 g

Fat: 10.45 g

Carbohydrates: 94.94 g

Breakfast Sausage and Mushroom Casserole

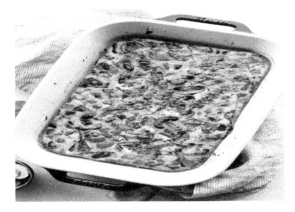

Preparation Time: 20 minutes

Cooking Time: 45 minutes

Servings: 4

Ingredients:

450g of Italian sausage, cooked and crumbled

Three-fourth cup of coconut milk

8 ounces of white mushrooms, sliced

1 medium onion, finely diced

2 Tablespoons of organic ghee

6 free-range eggs

600g of sweet potatoes

1 red bell pepper, roasted

3/4 tsp. of ground black pepper, divided

1 ½ tsp. of sea salt, divided

Directions:

Peel and shred the sweet potatoes.

Take a bowl, fill it with ice-cold water, and soak the sweet potatoes in it. Set aside.

Peel the roasted bell pepper, remove its seeds and finely dice it.

Set the oven 375°F.

Get a casserole baking dish and grease it with the organic ghee.

Put a skillet over medium flame and cook the mushrooms in it. Cook until the mushrooms are crispy and brown.

Take the mushrooms out and mix them with the crumbled sausage.

Now sauté the onions in the same skillet. Cook up to the onions are soft and golden. This should take about 4 – 5 minutes.

Take the onions out and mix them in the sausage-mushroom mixture.

Add the diced bell pepper to the same mixture.

Mix well and set aside for a while.

Now drain the soaked shredded potatoes, put them on a paper towel, and pat dry.

Bring the sweet potatoes in a bowl and add about a teaspoon of salt and half a teaspoon of ground black pepper to it. Mix well and set aside.

Now take a large bowl and crack the eggs in it.

Break the eggs and then blend in the coconut milk.

Stir in the remaining black pepper and salt.

Take the greased casserole dish and spread the seasoned sweet potatoes evenly in the base of the dish.

Next, spread the sausage mixture evenly in the dish.

Finally, spread the egg mixture.

Now cover the casserole dish using a piece of aluminum foil.

Bake for 20 - 30 minutes. To check if the casserole is baked properly, insert a tester in the middle of the casserole, and it should come out clean.

Uncover the casserole dish and bake it again, uncovered for 5 - 10 minutes, until the casserole is a little golden on the top.

Allow it to cool for 10 minutes.

Enjoy!

Nutrition:

Calories: 598 kcal

Protein: 28.65 g

Fat: 36.75 g

Carbohydrates: 48.01 g

Fennel Seeds Cookies

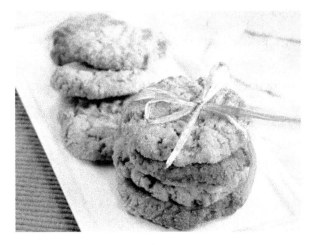

Preparation Time: 10 minutes

Cooking Time: 20 minutes

37

Servings: 5

Ingredients:

1/3 cup coconut flour

¼ teaspoon whole fennel seeds

½ teaspoon fresh ginger, grated finely

¼ cup coconut oil, softened

2 tablespoons raw honey

1 teaspoon vanilla extract

Pinch of ground cinnamon

Pinch of salt

Pinch freshly ground black pepper

Directions:

Set the oven to 360°F. Line a cookie sheet that has a parchment paper.

In a substantial bowl, add all together the ingredients and mix till an even dough form.

Form a small balls in the mixture make onto a prepared cookie sheet inside a single layer.

Using your fingers, gently press along the balls to create the cookies.

Bake for at least 9 minutes or till golden brown.

Nutrition:

Calories: 353

Fat: 5g

Carbohydrates: 19g

Fiber: 3g

Protein: 25g

Cinnamon-Apple Granola with Greek Yogurt

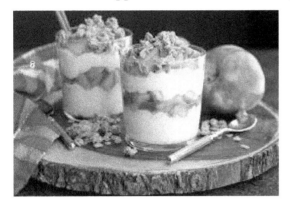

Preparation Time: 5 minutes

Cooking Time: 10 minutes

Servings: 2

Ingredients:

1/2 c. raw almonds, chopped (or raw nuts of choice)

1/2 c. raw walnuts, chopped (or raw nuts of choice)

1/2 apple, peeled and diced

1 tbsp. almond flour

2 tbsp. vanilla protein powder

1 tsp. ground cinnamon

1/8 c. applesauce, unsweetened preferred

2 tsp. honey

2 tsp. almond butter

1/16 tsp. vanilla extract

39

dash of sea salt

1 cup Greek plain or vanilla yogurt (or flavor of choice)

Directions:

In a mixing bowl, combine the chopped almonds, chopped walnuts (or preferred raw nuts), diced apple, vanilla protein powder, almond flour, lucuma (opt), and cinnamon and salt in a bowl. Mix well.

In a second bowl, combine the apple sauce, almond butter, honey, and vanilla extract. Mix well. Pour the bowl with the nuts into the bowl with the wet ingredients and blend together thoroughly. Make sure all dry ingredients get coated.

Place the granola mixture onto a parchment paper-lined baking sheet and bake until the desired crunch is obtained approximately 8 to 10 minutes. Take off from oven and let cool or eat hot. Place 1/2 cup each Greek yogurt into two bowls. Divide the granola and sprinkle over the yogurt in each bowl. Serve immediately.

Nutrition:

Calories: 312 kcal

Protein: 11.72 g

Fat: 22.37 g

Carbohydrates: 19.92 g

Banana-Oatmeal Vegan Pancakes

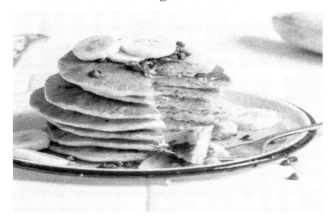

Preparation Time: 5 minutes

Cooking Time: 5 minutes

Servings: 12

Ingredients:

1¼ c. old fashioned oats

½ c. organic whole wheat flour

2 tsp. Baking powder

½ tsp. sea salt

1½ c. soymilk

2 ripe bananas

Directions:

To begin, heat griddle or skillet over medium heat.

Next, place all ingredients, except for banana, into a blender and process until smooth. Add the bananas to blender and blend until smooth.

Lightly grease griddle with olive or coconut oil, then pour ¼ c. of batter onto griddle and cook for at least 2 to 3 minutes, then flip and cook for about 2 minutes or up to the pancake is golden brown and cooked through.

Repeat process with remaining batter.

Nutrition:

Calories: 59 kcal

Protein: 3.49 g

Fat: 1.48 g

Carbohydrates: 11.52 g

Peanut Butter-Banana Muffins

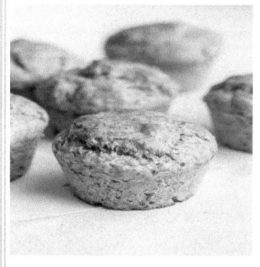

Preparation Time: 15 minutes

Cooking Time: 25 minutes

Servings: 12

Ingredients:

1½ c. all-purpose flour

1 c. old-fashioned oats

1 tsp. Baking powder

½ tsp. Baking soda

½ tsp. salt

2 tbsp. Applesauce

¾ c. light brown sugar

2 large eggs

1 c. mashed banana (about 3 bananas)

6 tbsp. creamy peanut butter

1 c. low-fat buttermilk

Directions:

Bring a small nonstick skillet on medium heat and spray lightly with cooking spray. Add in the bell pepper and onion and sauté for 1 to 2 minutes, or until both are tender and the onion translucent.

In a small bowl, crack in eggs and whisk. Add in milk; whisk until well-blended. Pour eggs into the pan and cook, frequently stirring until eggs are scrambled to your liking.

To serve, spoon half the egg mixture into each tortilla, wrap, and serve. Try serving with a side of fresh fruit for a complete meal.

Nutrition:

Calories: 187 kcal

Protein: 8.12 g

Fat: 6.25 g

Carbohydrates: 27.82 g

Bake Apple Turnover

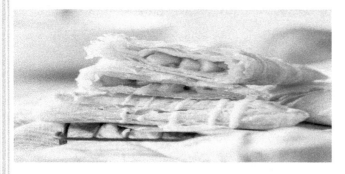

Preparation Time: 30 minutes

Cooking Time: 25 minutes

Servings: 4

Ingredients:

For the turnovers

4 apples, peeled, cored, diced into bite-sized pieces

1 Tbsp. almond flour

All-purpose flour, for rolling out the dough

1 frozen puff pastry, thawed

½ cup palm sugar, crumbled by hand to loosen granules

½ tsp. cinnamon powder

For the egg wash

1 egg white, whisked in

2 Tbsp. water

Directions:

For the filling: combine almond flour, cinnamon powder, and palm sugar until these resemble coarse meal. Toss in diced apples until well coated. Set aside.

On a lightly floured surface, roll the puff pastry until ¼ inch thin. Slice into 8 pieces of 4" x 4" squares.

Divide prepared apples into 8 equal portions. Spoon on individual puff pastry squares. Fold in half diagonally. Press edges to seal.

Place each filled pastry on a baking tray lined with parchment paper. Make sure there is ample space between pastries.

Freeze for at least 20 minutes, or till ready to bake.

Preheat oven to 400°F or 205°C for at 10 minutes.

Brush frozen pastries with egg wash. Bring in a hot oven, and cook for 12 to 15 minutes, or until these turn golden brown all over.

Take off the baking tray in the oven immediately. Cool slightly for easier handling.

Place 1 apple turnover on a plate. Serve warm.

Nutrition:

Calories: 203 kcal

Protein: 5.29 g

Fat: 4.4 g

Carbohydrates: 38.25 g

Quinoa and Cauliflower Congee

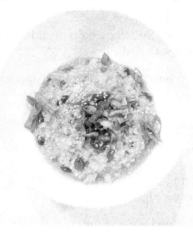

Preparation Time: 10 minutes

Cooking Time:1 hour

Servings: 8

Ingredients:

1 cauliflower head, minced

2 tablespoons red quinoa

2 leeks, minced

1 tablespoon fresh ginger, grated

2 garlic cloves, grated

6 cups of water

2 tablespoons brown rice

1 tablespoon olive oil

1 tablespoon fish sauce

2 onions, minced

Pinch of white pepper

For Garnish

4 eggs, soft-boiled

2 red chilli, minced

1 lime, sliced into wedges

¼ cup packed basil leaves, torn

¼ cup loosely packed cilantro leaves, torn

¼ cup loosely packed spearmint leaves, torn

Directions:

Put olive oil into a huge skillet on medium heat. Sauté shallots, garlic, and ginger until limp and aromatic; pour into a slow cooker set at medium heat.

Except for garnishes, pour remaining ingredients into slow cooker; stir. Put the lid on. Cook for 6 hours. Turn off heat. Taste; adjust seasoning if needed.

Ladle congee into individual bowls. Garnish with basil leaves, cilantro leaves, red chilli, and spearmint leaves. Add 1 piece of soft-boiled egg on top of each; serve with a wedge of lime on the side. Slice egg just before eating so yolk runs into congee. Squeeze lime juice into congee just before eating.

Nutrition:

Calories: 138 kcal

Protein: 7.23 g

Fat: 7.65 g

Carbohydrates: 10.76 g

Breakfast Arrozcaldo

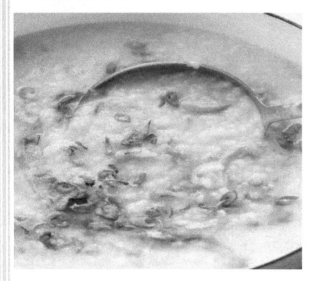

Preparation Time: 20 minutes

Cooking Time: 30 minutes

Servings: 5

Ingredients:

6 eggs, white only

1½ cups brown rice, cooked

For the filling

¼ cup raisins

½ cup frozen peas, thawed

1 white onion, minced

1 garlic clove, minced

oil, for greasing

Directions:

For the filling, spray a small amount of oil into a skillet set over medium heat. Add in onion and garlic. Stir-fry until former is limp and transparent.

Stir-fry while breaking up clumps, about 2 minutes. Add in remaining ingredients. Stir-fry for another minute.

Turn down the heat, and let filling cook for 10 to 15 minutes, or until juices are greatly reduced. Stir often. Turn off heat. Divide into 6 equal portions.

For the eggs, spray a small amount of oil into a smaller skillet set over medium heat. Cook eggs. Discard yolk. Transfer to holding the plate.

To serve, place 1 portion of rice on a plate, 1 portion of filling, and 1 egg white. Serve warm.

Nutrition:

Calories: 53 kcal

Protein: 6.28 g

Fat: 1.35 g

Carbohydrates: 3.59 g

Whole Grain Blueberry Scones

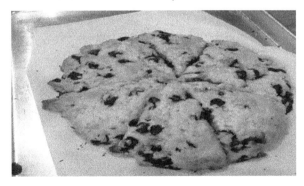

Preparation Time: 10 minutes

Cooking Time: 25 minutes

Servings: 8

Ingredients:

2 cups of whole-wheat flour

¼ cup maple syrup

6 tablespoons of olive oil

2-1/2 teaspoons baking powder

½ teaspoon sea salt

2 tablespoons of coconut milk

1 teaspoon vanilla extract

1 cup blueberries

Directions:

Set the oven 400°F. Keep parchment paper on your baking sheet.

Add the syrup, flour, salt, and baking powder in a bowl. Combine well by whisking together.

Pour the olive oil into a bowl with the dry ingredients.

Work the oil into your flour mix.

Stir the vanilla extract and coconut milk into the dry ingredients bowl.

Fold in the blueberries gently. Your dough should be sticky and thick.

Put some flour on your hand then shape the dough into a circle.

Take a knife and create triangle slices.

Keep them on the baking sheet. Maintain an 8-inch gap.

Bake for 25 minutes. Set aside on the baking sheet for cooling once done.

Nutrition:

Calories 331

Carbohydrates 27g

Cholesterol 0mg

Total Fat 23g

 Protein 4g

Fiber 4g

Sugar 8g

Tuna & Sweet Potato Croquettes

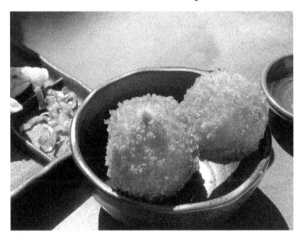

Preparation Time: 15 minutes

Cooking Time: 12 minutes

Servings: 8

Ingredients:

1 tablespoon coconut oil

½ large onion, chopped

1 (1-inch piece fresh ginger, minced

3 garlic cloves, minced

1 Serrano pepper, seeded and minced

½ teaspoon ground coriander

¼ teaspoon ground turmeric

¼ teaspoon red chili powder

¼ teaspoon garam masala

Salt, to taste

Freshly ground black pepper, to taste

2 (5 oz.) cans tuna

1 cup sweet potato, peeled and mashed

1 egg

¼ cup tapioca flour

¼ cup almond flour

Olive oil, as required

Directions:

In a frying pan, warm the coconut oil on medium heat.

Put onion, ginger, garlic, and Serrano pepper and sauté for approximately 5-6 minutes.

Stir in spices and sauté approximately 1 minute more.

Transfer the onion mixture in a bowl.

Add tuna and sweet potato and mix till well combined.

Make equal sized oblong shaped patties in the mixture.

Arrange the croquettes inside a baking sheet in a very single layer and refrigerate for overnight.

52

In a shallow dish, beat the egg.

In another shallow dish, mix together both flours.

In a big skillet, heat the enough oil.

Add croquettes in batches and shallow fry for around 2-3 minutes per side.

Nutrition:

Calories: 404

Fat: 9g

Carbohydrates: 20g

Fiber: 4g

Protein: 30g

Snacks , Sides and Appetizers

Green Beans

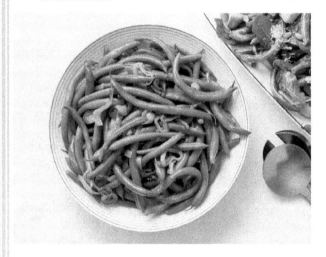

Preparation Time: 5 minutes

Cooking Time: 10 minutes

Servings: 5

Ingredients:

½ teaspoon of red pepper flakes

2 tablespoons of extra-virgin olive oil

2 garlic cloves, minced

1-1/2 lbs. green beans, trimmed

2 tablespoons of water

½ teaspoon kosher salt

Directions:

Heat oil in a skillet on medium temperature.

Include the pepper flake. Stir to coat in the olive oil.

Include the green beans. Cook for 7 minutes.

Stir often. The beans should be brown in some areas.

Add the salt and garlic. Cook for 1 minute, while stirring.

Pour water and cover immediately.

Cook covered for 1 more minute.

Nutrition:

Calories 82

Carbohydrates 6g

Total Fat 6g

Protein 1g

Fiber 2g

Sugar 0g

Sodium 230mg

Roasted Carrots

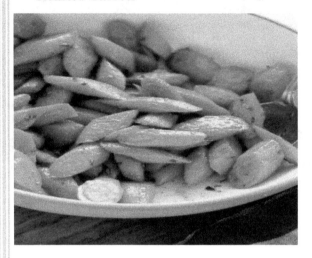

Preparation Time: 10 minutes

Cooking Time: 40 minutes

Servings: 4

Ingredients:

1 onion, peeled & cut

 8 carrots, peeled & cut

1 teaspoon thyme, chopped

2 tablespoons of extra-Moroccan Style Couscous

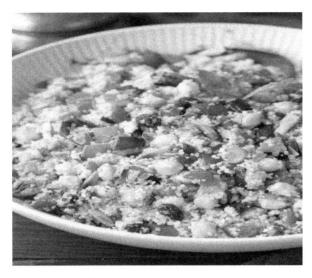

Preparation Time: 10 minutes

Cooking Time: 10 minutes

Servings: 4

Ingredients:

1 cup yellow couscous

½ teaspoon ground cardamom

1 cup chicken stock

1 tablespoon butter

1 teaspoon salt

½ teaspoon red pepper

Directions:

Toss butter in the pan and melt it.

Add couscous and roast it for 1 minute over the high heat.

Then add ground cardamom, salt, and red pepper. Stir it well.

57

Pour the chicken stock and bring the mixture to boil.

Simmer couscous for 5 minutes with the closed lid.

Nutrition:

Calories 196

Fat 3.4g

Fiber 2.4g

Carbs 35g

Protein 5.9g

Creamy Polenta

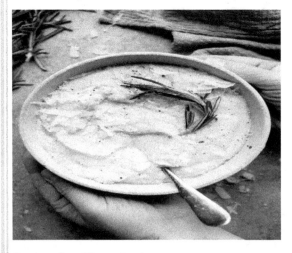

Preparation Time: 8 minutes

Cooking Time: 45 minutes

Servings: 4

Ingredients:

1 cup polenta

1 ½ cup water

2 cups chicken stock

½ cup cream

1/3 cup Parmesan, grated

Directions:

Put polenta in the pot.

Add water, chicken stock, cream, and Parmesan. Mix up polenta well.

Then preheat oven to 355F.

Cook polenta in the oven for 45 minutes.

Mix up the cooked meal with the help of the spoon carefully before serving.

Nutrition:

Calories 208

Fat 5.3g

Fiber 1g

Carbs 32.2g

Protein 8g

Mushroom Millet

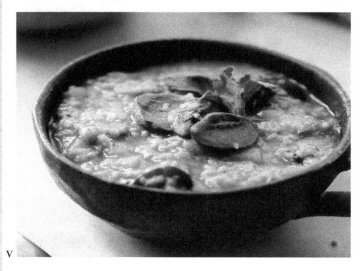

v

Preparation Time: 10 minutes

Cooking Time: 15 minutes

Servings: 3

Ingredients:

¼ cup mushrooms, sliced

¾ cup onion, diced

1 tablespoon olive oil

1 teaspoon salt

3 tablespoons milk

½ cup millet

1 cup of water

1 teaspoon butter

Directions:

Pour olive oil in the skillet then put the onion.

Add mushrooms and roast the vegetables for 10 minutes over the medium heat. Stir them from time to time.

Meanwhile, pour water in the pan.

Add millet and salt.

Cook the millet with the closed lid for 15 minutes over the medium heat.

Then add the cooked mushroom mixture in the millet.

Add milk and butter. Mix up the millet well.

Nutrition:

Calories 198

Fat 7.7g

Fiber 3.5g

Carbs 27.9g

Protein 4.7g

Spicy Barley

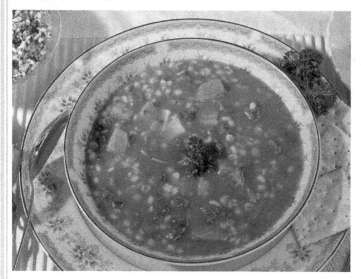

Preparation Time: 7 minutes

Cooking Time: 42 minutes

Servings: 5

Ingredients:

1 cup barley

3 cups chicken stock

½ teaspoon cayenne pepper

1 teaspoon salt

½ teaspoon chili pepper

½ teaspoon ground black pepper

1 teaspoon butter

1 teaspoon olive oil

Directions:

Place barley and olive oil in the pan.

Roast barley on high heat for 1 minute. Stir it well.

Then add salt, chili pepper, ground black pepper, cayenne pepper, and butter.

Add chicken stock.

Close the lid and cook barley for 40 minutes over the medium-low heat.

Nutrition:

Calories 152

Fat 2.9g

Fiber 6.5g

Carbs 27.8g

Protein 5.1g

Couscous Salad

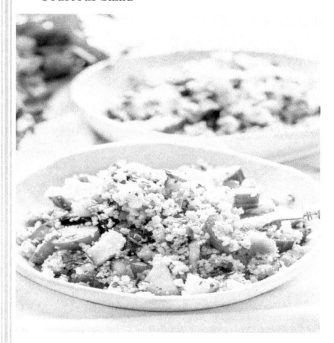

Preparation Time: 10 minutes

Cooking Time: 6 minutes

Servings: 4

Ingredients:

1/3 cup couscous

1/3 cup chicken stock

¼ teaspoon ground black pepper

¾ teaspoon ground coriander

½ teaspoon salt

¼ teaspoon paprika

¼ teaspoon turmeric

1 tablespoon butter

2 oz. chickpeas, canned, drained

1 cup fresh arugula, chopped

2 oz. sun-dried tomatoes, chopped

1 oz. Feta cheese, crumbled

1 tablespoon canola oil

Directions:

Bring the chicken stock to boil.

Add couscous, ground black pepper, ground coriander, salt, paprika, and turmeric. Add chickpeas and butter. Stir the mixture well and close the lid.

Let the couscous soak the hot chicken stock for 6 minutes.

Meanwhile, in the mixing bowl combine together arugula, sun-dried tomatoes, and Feta cheese.

Add cooked couscous mixture and canola oil.

Mix up the salad well.

Nutrition:

Calories 18

Fat 9g

Fiber 3.6g

Carbs 21.1g

Protein 6g

Cauliflower Broccoli Mash

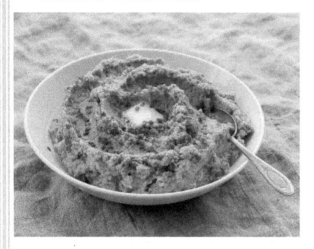

Preparation Time: 5 minutes

Cooking Time: 10 minutes

Serving: 6

Ingredients:

1 large head cauliflower, cut into chunks

1 small head broccoli, cut into florets

3 tablespoons extra virgin olive oil

1 teaspoon salt

Pepper, to taste

Directions:

Take a pot and add oil then heat it

Add the cauliflower and broccoli

Season with salt and pepper to taste

Keep stirring to make vegetable soft

Add water if needed

When is already cooked, use a food processor or a potato masher to puree the vegetables

Serve and enjoy!

Nutrition:

Calories: 39

Fat: 3g

Carbohydrates: 2g

Protein: 0.89g

Brussels Sprout Chips

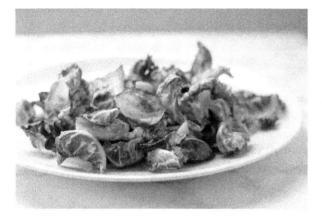

Preparation Time: 10 minutes

Cooking Time: 10 minutes

Servings: 4

Ingredients:

2 cups Brussels sprout leaves

2 tablespoons ghee

Kosher salt

Lemon zest

Directions:

Set the oven to 350F, then cover two cookie sheets with parchment paper.

Put the leaves in a huge bowl and pour melted ghee over the top, and add salt.

Bake for at least 8 to 10 minutes or until the leaves are crispy. If they are soft at all, put them back in the oven.

While still hot, sprinkle the lemon zest over the leaves. Serve warm.

Nutrition:

Calories: 42 kcal

Protein: 3.13 g

Fat: 1.68 g

Carbohydrates: 4.77 g

Cauliflower Snacks

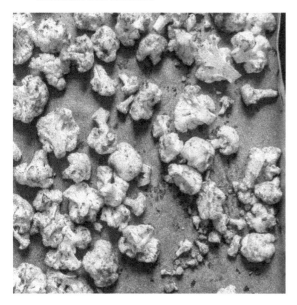

Preparation Time: 10 minutes

Cooking Time: 60 minutes

Servings: 4

Ingredients:

1 head of cauliflower

4 tablespoons extra virgin olive oil

1 teaspoon salt

Directions:

Set the oven to 425F, then prepare two cookie sheets by lining them with parchment paper.

Trim off the cauliflower florets and discard the core. Cut the florets into golf-ball-sized pieces.

69

Place the cauliflower in a bowl, and pour olive oil over them and sprinkle with salt. Mix to coat. Spread in a single layer, not touching.

Roast about 1 hour, turning the cauliflower three to four times until golden brown. Serve warm.

Nutrition:

Calories: 91 kcal

Protein: 2.93 g

Fat: 7.7 g

Carbohydrates: 3.29 g

virgin olive oil

½ teaspoon rosemary, chopped

¼ teaspoon ground pepper

½ teaspoon salt

Directions:

Preheat your oven to 425 degrees F.

Mix the onions and carrots by tossing in a bowl with rosemary, thyme, pepper, and salt. Spread on your baking sheet.

Roast for 40 minutes. The onions and carrots should be browning and tender.

Nutrition:

Calories 126

Carbohydrates 16g

Total Fat 6g

Protein 2g

Fiber 4g

Sugar 8g

Sodium 286mg

Tomato Bulgur

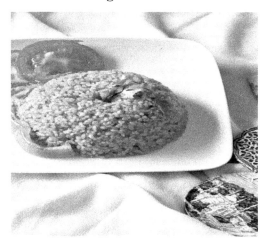

Preparation Time: 7 minutes

Cooking Time: 20 minutes

Servings: 2

Ingredients:

½ cup bulgur

1 teaspoon tomato paste

½ white onion, diced

2 tablespoons coconut oil

1 ½ cup chicken stock

Directions:

Toss coconut oil in the pan and melt it.

Add diced onion and roast it until light brown.

71

Then add bulgur and stir well.

Cook bulgur in coconut oil for 3 minutes.

Then add tomato paste and mix up bulgur until homogenous.

Add chicken stock.

Close the lid and cook bulgur for 15 minutes over the medium heat.

The cooked bulgur should soak all liquid.

Nutrition:

Calories 257

Fat 14.5g

Fiber 7.1g

Carbs 30.2g

Protein 5.2g

Cucumber Yogurt

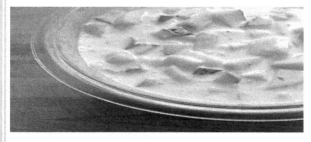

Preparation Time: 5 minutes

Cooking Time: 0 minutes

Servings: 1

Ingredients:

1 cup cucumbers, skin removed and chopped in chunks

2 tablespoons chopped cashews

1/4 cup fat-free Greek yogurt

2 teaspoons fresh-squeezed lemon juice

1 teaspoon fresh dill, chopped fine

Directions:

Peel and chop the cucumbers, then place them in a bowl.

Add the cashews, yogurt, lemon juice, and dill.

Mix well, grab a spoon, and enjoy.

Nutrition:

Calories: 300 kcal

Protein: 11.35 g

Fat: 23.55 g

Carbohydrates: 14.13 g

Hummus Deviled Eggs

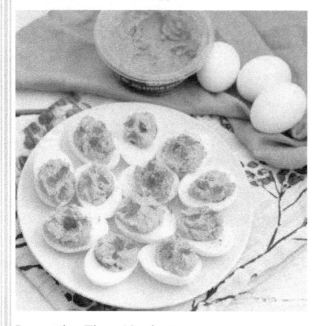

Preparation Time: 10 minutes

Cooking Time: 0 minutes

Servings: 6

Ingredients:

6 hard-boiled eggs

1/2 cup hummus

Paprika

Directions:

Slice the hardboiled eggs in half lengthwise and remove the yolk.

Fill the egg whites with hummus and sprinkle with paprika before serving.

Nutrition:

74

Calories: 179 kcal

Protein: 11.03 g

Fat: 12.41 g

Carbohydrates: 5.14 g

Hummus with Celery

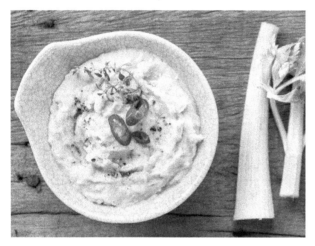

Preparation Time: 15 minutes

Cooking Time: 0 minutes

Servings: 4

Ingredients:

1/4 cup lemon juice

1/4 cup tahini

3 cloves of garlic, crushed

2 tablespoons extra virgin olive oil

1/2 teaspoon salt

1/2 teaspoon cumin

1 (15–ounce) can chickpeas

2 to 3 tablespoons water

Dash of paprika

6 stalks celery, cut into 2-inch pieces

3 tablespoons salsa

Directions:

Using a food processor mix the lemon juice and tahini for about a minute, until it is smooth. Scrape the sides down and process for 30 more seconds.

Add the garlic, olive oil, salt, and cumin. Blend for about 1 minute.

Drain the chickpeas, put the half of them on the food processor, and blend for another minute. Scrape down the sides, add the other half of the chickpeas, and process until smooth, about 2 minutes. If it like a little too thick, add water, 1 tablespoon at a time until you reach the desired consistency.

Fill the celery sticks with hummus and sprinkle paprika on top.

Serve with salsa for dipping.

Nutrition:

Calories: 240 kcal

Protein: 9.27 g

Fat: 14.51 g

Carbohydrates: 21.01 g

Kale Chips

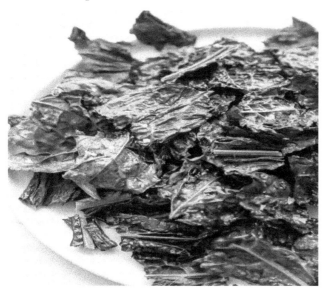

Preparation Time: 10 minutes

Cooking Time: 2 hours

Servings: 8

Ingredients:

2 bunches of curly kale with stems removed, washed and torn into bite-sized pieces

1 cup grated sweet potato

1 cup cashews, soaked and softened in water about 2 hours

2 tablespoons nutritional yeast (found at health food stores)

The juice of 1 lemon

2 tablespoons honey

1/2 teaspoon sea salt

2 tablespoons water

Directions:

Put the kale in a huge bowl and set aside.

In a blender or food processor, process the sweet potato, softened cashews yeast, lemon juice, honey, salt, and water until smooth. Put the mixture on the kale and toss with your hands to coat the leaves.

Spread the kale leaves out on a large cookie sheet in a single layer without touching.

Set the oven to its lowest setting.

Prop the oven door slightly ajar and dehydrate the chips for about 2 hours, turning the cookie sheet and watching to make sure the chips do not burn.

When crisp, remove from the oven and let cool. Store in an airtight container.

Nutrition:

Calories: 40 kcal

Protein: 2.19 g

Fat: 0.87 g

Carbohydrates: 6.39 g

Fresh Strawberry Salsa

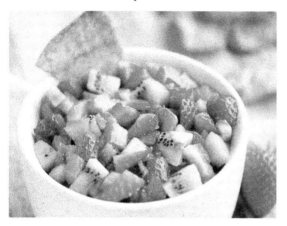

Preparation Time: 10 minutes

Cooking Time: 0 minutes

Servings: 6-8

Ingredients:

½ teaspoon lime zest, grated

2 teaspoons pure raw honey

2 kiwi fruit, peeled, chopped

½ cup fresh cilantro

¼ cup fresh lime juice

2 pounds fresh ripe strawberries, hulled, chopped

½ cup red onion, finely chopped

1-2 jalapeños, deseeded, finely chopped

Directions:

Add lime juice, lime zest and honey into a large bowl and whisk well.

79

Add rest of the ingredients then mix well. Cover and set aside for a while for the flavors to set in. Serve.

Nutrition:

Calories: 119 kcal

Protein: 9.26 g

Fat: 4.38 g

Carbohydrates: 11.73 g

Mini Pepper Nachos

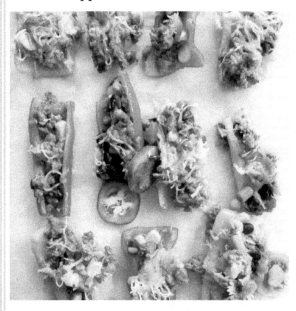

Preparation Time: 5 minutes

Cooking Time: 10 minutes

Servings: 8

Ingredients:

.5 cup Tomato, chopped

1 tbsp. Chili powder

1.5 cup Cheddar cheese, shredded

1 tsp. Cumin, ground

16 oz. Mini peppers, seeded, halved

1 tsp. Garlic powder

16 oz. Ground beef

1 tsp. Paprika

.25 tsp. Red pepper flakes

5 tsp. Salt

.5 tsp. Oregano

5 tsp. Pepper

Directions:

Mix seasonings together in a bowl.

On medium heat, brown the meat, be sure all the clumps are broken up.

Mix in the spices and continue to sauté until the seasoning has gone through all of the meat.

Heat the oven to 400F.

Place the peppers in a single line. They can touch.

Coat with the beef mix.

Sprinkle with cheese.

Bake for at least 10 minutes or until cheese has melted.

Pull out of the oven and top with the toppings.

Nutrition:

Calories: 240 kcal

Protein: 11.01 g

Fat: 18.2 g

Carbohydrates: 9.49 g

Avocado Hummus

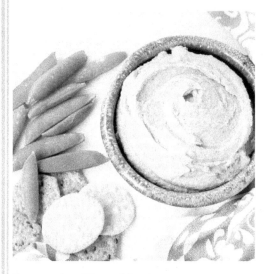

Preparation Time: 15 minutes

Cooking Time: 0 minutes

Servings: 4

Ingredients:

.25 tsp. Pepper

.5 tsp. Salt

5 tsp. Cumin

1 clove pressed garlic

.5 Lemon juice

.25 cup Tahini

.25 cup Sunflower seeds

.5 cup Coconut oil

.5 cup Cilantro

3 Avocados

Directions:

Halve the avocados, take off the pits, then spoon out the flesh.

Put all together ingredients in a blender and mix until completely smooth.

Add water, lemon juice, or oil if you need to loosen the mixture bit.

Nutrition:

Calories: 651 kcal

Protein: 9.62 g

Fat: 64.05 g

Carbohydrates: 19.95 g

Flavorsome Almonds

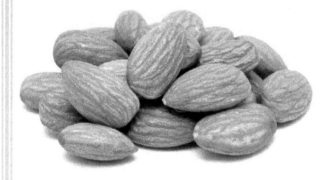

Preparation Time: 10 minutes

Cooking Time: 15 minutes

Servings: 8

Ingredients:

2 cups of whole almonds

3 tbsp. of raw honey

1 tsp. of extra-virgin olive oil

1 tbsp. of filtered water

½ tsp. of chili powder

½ tsp. of ground cinnamon

¼ tsp. of ground cumin

¼ tsp. of cayenne pepper

Salt, to taste

Directions:

Preheat the oven to 350 degrees F.

Arrange the almonds onto a large rimmed baking sheet in a single layer.

Roast for about 10 minutes.

Meanwhile, in a microwave-safe bowl, add honey and microwave on Hugh for about 30 seconds.

Remove from microwave and stir in oil and water.

In a small bowl, mix together all spices.

Remove the almonds from the oven, add it into the bowl of honey mixture, and stir to combine well.

Transfer the almond mixture onto the baking sheet in a single layer.

Sprinkle with spice mixture evenly.

Roast for about 3-4 minutes.

Take off from oven and keep aside to cool completely before serving.

You can preserve these roasted almonds in an airtight jar.

Nutrition:

Calories: 168

Fat: 12.5g

Carbs: 11.8g

Protein: 5.1g

Fiber: 3.1g

Cool Garbanzo and Spinach Beans

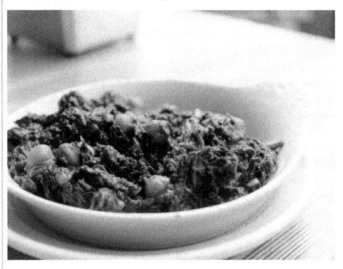

Preparation Time: 5-10 minutes

Cooking Time: 0 minute

Serving: 4

Ingredients:

12 ounces garbanzo beans

1 tablespoon olive oil

½ onion, diced

½ teaspoon cumin

10 ounces spinach, chopped

Directions:

Take a skillet and add olive oil

Place it over medium-low heat

Add onions, garbanzo and cook for 5 minutes

Stir in cumin, garbanzo beans, spinach and season with sunflower seeds

Use a spoon to smash gently

Cook thoroughly

Serve and enjoy!

Nutrition:

Calories: 90

Fat: 4g

Carbohydrates:11g

Protein:4g

Onion and Orange Healthy Salad

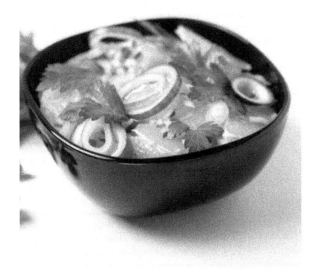

Preparation Time: 10 minutes

Cooking Time: 0 minutes

Serving: 3

Ingredients:

6 large orange

3 tablespoon of red wine vinegar

6 tablespoon of olive oil

1 teaspoon of dried oregano

1 red onion, thinly sliced

1 cup olive oil

¼ cup of fresh chives, chopped

Ground black pepper

Directions:

Peel the orange and cut each of them in 4-5 crosswise slices

Transfer the oranges to a shallow dish

Drizzle vinegar, olive oil and sprinkle oregano

Toss

Chill for 30 minutes

Arrange sliced onion and black olives on top

Decorate with an additional sprinkle of chives and a fresh grind of pepper

Serve and enjoy!

Nutrition:

Calories: 120

Fat: 6g

Carbohydrates: 20g

Protein: 2g

Stir-Fried Almond And Spinach

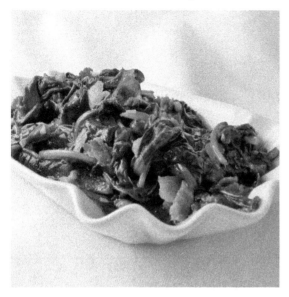

Preparation Time: 10 minutes

Cooking Time: 15 minutes

Serving: 2

Ingredients:

34 pounds spinach

3 tablespoons almonds

Salt to taste

1 tablespoon coconut oil

Directions:

Put oil to a large pot and place it on high heat

Add spinach and let it cook, stirring frequently

Once the spinach is cooked and tender, season with salt and stir

Add almonds and enjoy!

Nutrition:

Calories: 150

Fat: 12g

Carbohydrates: 10g

Protein: 8g

Cilantro And Avocado Platter

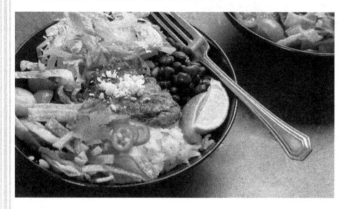

Preparation Time: 10 minutes

Cooking Time: 0 minutes

Serving: 6

Ingredients:

2 avocados, peeled, pitted and diced

1 sweet onion, chopped

1 green bell pepper, chopped

1 large ripe tomato, chopped

¼ cup of fresh cilantro, chopped

½ a lime, juiced

Salt and pepper as needed

Directions:

Take a medium-sized bowl and add onion, bell pepper, tomato, avocados, lime and cilantro

Mix well and give it a toss

Season with salt and pepper according to your taste

Serve and enjoy!

Nutrition:

Calories: 126

Fat: 10g

Carbohydrates: 10g

Protein: 2g

Lunch

Shrimp with Cinnamon Sauce

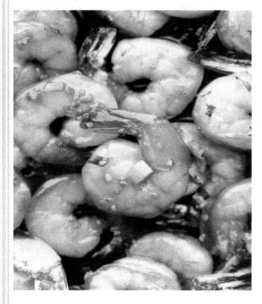

Preparation Time: 10 minutes

Cooking Time: 10 minutes

Servings: 4

Ingredients:

2 tbsp. Extra Virgin Olive Oil

1½ Pound Peeled Shrimp

2 tbsp. Dijon Mustard

1 cup No Salt Added Chicken Broth

1 tsp. Ground Cinnamon

1 tsp. Onion Powder

½ tsp. Sea Salt

¼ tsp. Freshly Ground Black Pepper

Directions:

In a huge nonstick skillet at medium-high heat, heat the olive oil until it shimmers.

Add the shrimp. Cook for at least 4 minutes, occasionally stirring, until the shrimp is opaque.

In a small bowl, whisk the mustard, chicken broth, cinnamon, onion powder, salt, and pepper. Pour this into the skillet and continue to cook for 3 minutes, stirring occasionally.

Nutrition:

Calories: 270

Total Fat: 11g

Total Carbs: 4g

Sugar: 1g

Fiber: 1g

Protein: 39g

Sodium: 664mg

Pan-Seared Scallops with Lemon-Ginger Vinaigrette

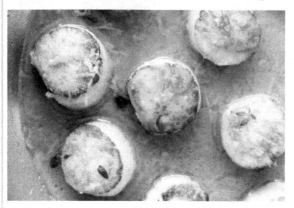

Preparation Time: 10 minutes

Cooking Time: 7 minutes

Servings: 4

Ingredients:

2 tbsp. Extra Virgin Olive Oil

1½ Pound Sea Scallop

½ tsp. Sea Salt

⅛ tsp. Freshly Ground Black Pepper

¼ cup Lemon Ginger Vinaigrette

Directions:

In a huge nonstick skillet at medium-high heat, heat the olive oil until it shimmers.

Season the scallops with pepper and salt and add them to the skillet. Cook for at least 3 minutes per side until just opaque.

Serve with the vinaigrette spooned over the top.

Nutrition:

Calories: 280

Total Fat: 16

Total Carbs: 5g

Sugar: 1g

 Fiber: 0g

Protein: 29g

Sodium: 508mg

Easy Crunchy Fish Tray Bake

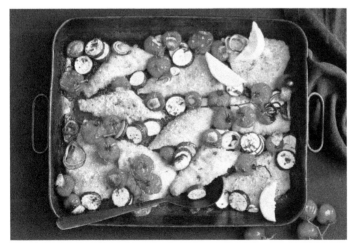

Preparation Time: 10 minutes

Cooking Time: 20 minutes

Servings: 4

Ingredients:

600g frozen crumbed whiting fish fillets

1/2 small red onion

2 x 250g punnets tomatoes

2 zucchini

180g baby stuffed peppers

1 tablespoon parmesan

2 teaspoons oregano leaves

1 lemon, cut into wedges

Directions:

Preheat the stove to 400F. Oil an enormous preparing plate. Spot the fish filets on the readied plate. Disperse the oregano & parmesan over the fish.

Add the zucchini, tomatoes & stuffed peppers to the plate. Disperse the onion rings over the top. Season well. Splash with olive oil. Heat until the fish is brilliant & cooked through.

Divide the fish & vegetables among plates & present with the rocket & lemon wedges.

Nutrition:

Calories: 346 kcal

Protein: 3.67 g

Fat: 2.8 g

Carbohydrates: 81.77 g

Ginger & Chili Sea Bass Fillets

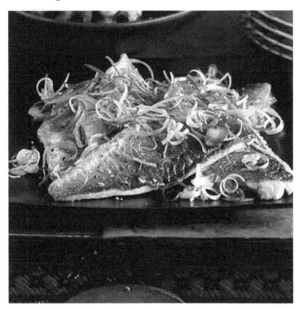

Preparation Time: 5 minutes

Cooking Time: 10 minutes

Servings: 2

Ingredients:

2 Sea bass fillet

1 tsp. Black pepper

1 tbsp. Extra virgin olive oil

1 tsp Ginger, peeled and chopped

1 Garlic cloves, thinly slice

1 Red chili, deseeded and thinly sliced

2 Green onion stemmed, chopped

97

Directions:

Get a skillet and heat the oil on a medium to high heat.

Sprinkle black pepper over the Sea Bass and score the fish's skin a few times with a sharp knife.

Add the sea bass fillet to the very hot pan with the skin side down.

Cook for 5 minutes and turn over.

Cook for a further 2 minutes.

Remove seabass from the pan and rest.

Put the chili, garlic, and ginger and cook for approximately 2 minutes or until golden.

Remove from the heat and add the green onions.

Scatter the vegetables over your sea bass to serve.

Try with a steamed sweet potato or side salad.

Nutrition:

Calories: 306 kcal

Protein: 29.92 g

Fat: 8.94 g

Carbohydrates: 26.59 g

Lemon & Garlic Chicken Thighs

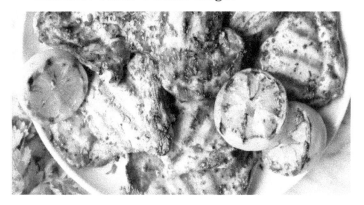

Preparation Time: 15 minutes

Cooking Time: 7 to 8 hours

Servings: 4

Ingredients:

2 cups chicken broth

1½ teaspoons garlic powder

1 teaspoon sea salt

Juice and zest of 1 large lemon

2 pounds boneless skinless chicken thighs

Directions:

Pour the broth into the slow cooker.

In a small bowl, put the garlic powder, salt, lemon juice, and lemon zest then stir. Baste each chicken thigh with an even coating of the mixture. Place the thighs along the bottom of the slow cooker.

Cover the cooker and set to low. Cook for around 7 to 8 hours, or until the internal temperature of the chicken reaches 165°F on a meat thermometer and the juices run clear, and serve.

99

Nutrition:

Calories: 29

Total Fat: 14g

Total Carbs: 3g

Sugar: 0g

Fiber: 0g

Protein: 43g

 Sodium: 1,017mg

White Bean, Chicken & Apple Cider Chili

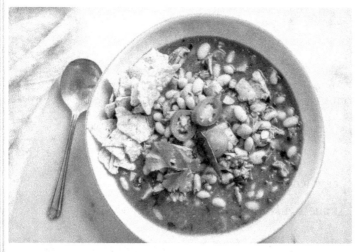

Preparation Time: 15 minutes

Cooking Time: 7 to 8 hours

Servings: 4

Ingredients:

3 cups chopped cooked chicken (see Basic "Rotisserie" Chicken)

2 (15-ounce) cans white navy beans, rinsed well and drained

1 medium onion, chopped

1 (15-ounce) can diced tomatoes

3 cups Chicken Bone Broth or store-bought chicken broth

1 cup apple cider

2 bay leaves

1 tablespoon extra-virgin olive oil

2 teaspoons garlic powder

1 teaspoon chili powder

1 teaspoon sea salt

½ teaspoon ground cumin

¼ teaspoon ground cinnamon

Pinch cayenne pepper

Freshly ground black pepper

¼ cup apple cider vinegar

Directions:

In your slow cooker, combine the chicken, beans, onion, tomatoes, broth, cider, bay leaves, olive oil, garlic powder, chili powder, salt, cumin, cinnamon cayenne, and season with black pepper.

Cover the cooker and set to low. Cook for 7 to 8 hours.

Remove and discard the bay leaves. Stir in the apple cider vinegar until well blended and serve.

Nutrition:

Calories: 469

Total Fat: 8g

Total Carbs: 46g

Sugar: 13g

Fiber: 9g

Protein: 51g

Sodium: 1,047mg

Pork with Olives

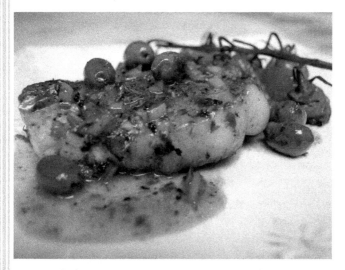

Preparation Time: 10 minutes

Cooking Time: 40 minutes

Servings: 4

Ingredients:

1 yellow onion, chopped

4 pork chops

2 tablespoons olive oil

1 tablespoon sweet paprika

2 tablespoons balsamic vinegar

¼ cup kalamata olives, pitted and chopped

1 tablespoon cilantro, chopped

Pinch of Sea Salt

Pinch black pepper

Directions:

Warm a pan with the oil on medium heat; add the onion and sauté for 5 minutes.

Add the meat and brown for a further 5 minutes.

Put the rest of the ingredients, toss, cook over medium heat for 30 minutes, divide between plates and serve.

Nutrition:

Calories 280

Fat 11g

Fiber 6g

Carbs 10g

Protein 21g

Pork Chops with Tomato Salsa

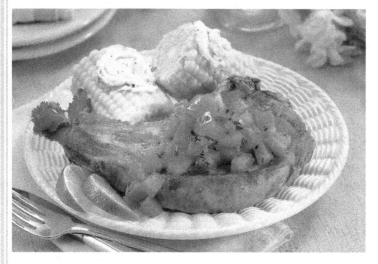

Preparation Time: 10 minutes

Cooking Time: 15 minutes

Servings: 4

Ingredients:

4 pork chops

1 tablespoon olive oil

4 scallions, chopped

1 teaspoon cumin, ground

½ tablespoon hot paprika

1 teaspoon garlic powder

Pinch of sea salt

Pinch of black pepper

1 small red onion, chopped

104

2 tomatoes, cubed

2 tablespoons lime juice

1 jalapeno, chopped

¼ cup cilantro, chopped

1 tablespoon lime juice

Directions:

Warm a pan with the oil on medium heat, add the scallions and sauté for 5 minutes.

Add the meat, cumin paprika, garlic powder, salt, and pepper, toss, cook for 5 minutes on each side, and divide between plates.

In a bowl, combine the tomatoes with the remaining ingredients, toss, divide next to the pork chops and serve.

Nutrition:

Calories 313

Fat 23.7g

Fiber 1.7g

Carbs 5.9g

Protein 19.2g

Mustard Pork Mix

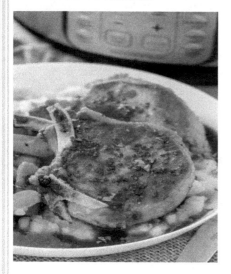

Preparation Time: 10 minutes

Cooking Time: 35 minutes

Servings: 4

Ingredients:

2 shallots, chopped

1 pound pork stew meat, cubed

2 garlic cloves, minced

2 tablespoons olive oil

¼ cup Dijon mustard

2 tablespoons chives, chopped

1 teaspoon cumin, ground

1 teaspoon rosemary, dried

Pinch of sea salt

Pinch black pepper

Directions:

Warm a pan with the oil on medium-high heat, add the shallots and sauté for 5 minutes.

Put the meat and brown for a further 5 minutes.

Put the rest of the ingredients, toss, cook on medium heat for 25 minutes more.

Divide the mix between plates and serve.

Nutrition:

Calories 280

Fat 14.3g

Fiber 6g

Carbs 11.8g

Protein 17g

Shrimp Scampi

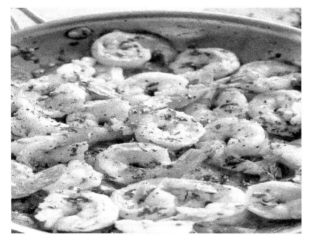

Preparation Time: 10 minutes

Cooking Time: 15 minutes

Servings: 4

Ingredients:

¼ cup Extra Olive Oil

1 Onion, Finely Chopped

1 Red Bell Pepper, Chopped

1½ Pound Shrimp, Peeled and Tails Removed

6 Garlic Cloves, Minced

2 Lemon Juices

2 Lemon Zest

½ tsp. Sea Salt

⅛ tsp. Freshly Ground Black Pepper

Directions:

In a huge nonstick skillet on medium-high heat, warm the olive oil until it shimmers.

Add the onion and red bell pepper. Cook for about 6 minutes, occasionally stirring, until soft.

Add the shrimp and cook for about 5 minutes until pink.

Add the garlic. Cook for 30 seconds, stirring constantly.

Add the lemon juice and zest, salt, and pepper. Simmer for 3 minutes.

Nutrition:

Calories: 345

Total Fat: 16

Total Carbs: 10g

Sugar: 3g

Fiber: 1g

Protein: 40g

Sodium: 424mg

Shrimp with Spicy Spinach

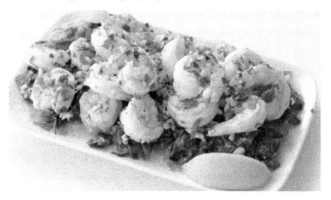

Preparation Time: 10 minutes

Cooking Time: 15 minutes

Servings: 4

Ingredients:

¼ cup Extra Olive Oil. divided

1½ Pound Peeled Shrimp

1 tsp. Sea Salt, divided

4 cups Baby fresh Spinach

6 Garlic cloves, minced

½ cup Freshly Squeezed Orange Juice

1 tbsp. Sriracha Sauce

⅛ tsp. Freshly ground black pepper

Directions:

In a huge nonstick skillet on medium-high heat, heat 2 tablespoons of the olive oil until it shimmers.

Add the shrimp and ½ teaspoon salt. Cook for at least 4 minutes, occasionally stirring, until the shrimp are pink. Transfer the shrimp to a plate, tent with aluminum foil to keep warm, and set aside.

Put back the skillet to the heat and heat the remaining 2 tablespoons of olive oil until it shimmers.

Add the spinach. Cook for 3 minutes, stirring.

Add the garlic. Cook for 30 seconds, stirring constantly.

In a small bowl, put and mix together the orange juice, Sriracha, remaining ½ teaspoon of salt, and pepper. Add this to the spinach and cook for 3 minutes. Serve the shrimp with the spinach on the side.

Nutrition:

Calories: 317

Total Fat: 16

Total Carbs: 7g

Sugar: 3

Fiber: 1g

Protein: 38g

Sodium: 911mg

Pork with Chili Zucchinis and Tomatoes

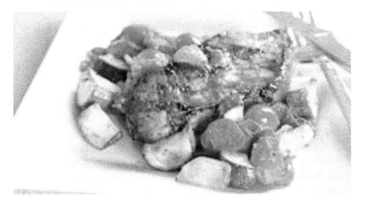

Preparation Time: 10 minutes

Cooking Time: 35 minutes

Servings: 4

Ingredients:

2 tomatoes, cubed

2 pounds pork stew meat, cubed

4 scallions, chopped

2 tablespoons olive oil

1 zucchini, sliced

Juice of 1 lime

2 tablespoons chili powder

½ tablespoons cumin powder

Pinch of sea salt

Pinch black pepper

Directions:

Warm a pan with the oil on medium heat, add the scallions and sauté for 5 minutes.

Add the meat and brown for 5 minutes more.

Add the tomatoes and the other ingredients, toss, cook over medium heat for 25 minutes more, divide between plates and serve.

Nutrition:

Calories 300

Fat 5g

Fiber 2g

Carbs 12g

Protein 14g

Pork with Thyme Sweet Potatoes

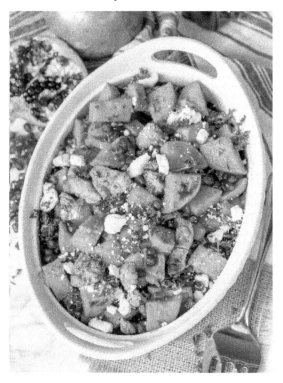

Preparation Time: 10 minutes

Cooking Time: 35 minutes

Servings: 4

Ingredients:

2 sweet potatoes, cut into wedges

4 pork chops

3 spring onions, chopped

1 tablespoon thyme, chopped

2 tablespoons olive oil

113

4 garlic cloves, minced

Pinch of sea salt

Pinch black pepper

½ cup vegetable stock

½ tablespoon chives, chopped

Directions:

In a roasting pan, combine the pork chops with the potatoes and the other ingredients, toss gently and cook at 390 degrees F for 35 minutes.

Divide everything between plates and serve.

Nutrition:

Calories 210

Fat 12.2g

Fiber 5.2g

Carbs 12g

Protein 10g

Parsley Pork and Artichokes

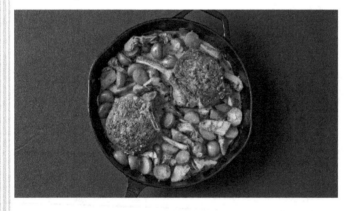

Preparation Time: 10 minutes

Cooking Time: 35 minutes

Servings: 4

Ingredients:

2 tbsp. balsamic vinegar

1 cup canned artichoke hearts, drained

2 tbsp. olive oil

2 lb. pork stew meat, cubed

2 tbsp. parsley, chopped

1 tsp. cumin, ground

1 tsp. turmeric powder

2 garlic cloves, minced

Pinch of sea salt

Pinch black pepper

Directions:

Warm a pan with the oil on medium heat, add the meat and brown for 5 minutes.

Add the artichokes, the vinegar, and the other ingredients, toss, cook over medium heat for 30 minutes, divide between plates and serve.

Nutrition:

Calories 260

Fat 5g

Fiber 4g

Carbs 11g

Protein 20g

Pork with Mushrooms and Cucumbers

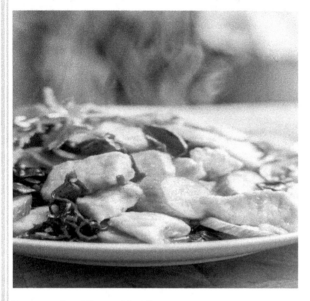

Preparation Time: 10 minutes

Cooking Time: 25 minutes

Servings: 4

Ingredients:

2 tablespoons olive oil

½ teaspoon oregano, dried

4 pork chops

2 garlic cloves, minced

Juice of 1 lime

¼ cup cilantro, chopped

Pinch of sea salt

116

Pinch black pepper

1 cup white mushrooms, halved

2 tablespoons balsamic vinegar

Directions:

Warm a pan with the oil on medium heat, add the pork chops and brown for 2 minutes on each side.

Put the rest of the ingredients, toss, cook on medium heat for 20 minutes, divide between plates and serve.

Nutrition:

Calories 220

Fat 6g

Fiber 8g

Carbs 14.2g

Protein 20g

Oregano Pork

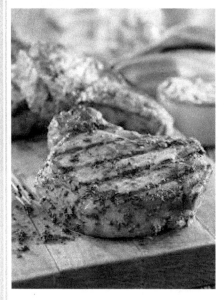

Preparation Time: 10 minutes

Cooking Time: 8 hours

Servings: 4

Ingredients:

2 pounds pork roast, sliced

2 tablespoons oregano, chopped

¼ cup balsamic vinegar

1 cup tomato paste

1 tablespoon sweet paprika

1 teaspoon onion powder

2 tablespoons chili powder

2 garlic cloves, minced

A pinch of salt and black pepper

Directions:

In your slow cooker, combine the roast with the oregano, the vinegar, and the other ingredients, toss, put the lid on and cook on Low for 8 hours.

Divide everything between plates and serve.

Nutrition:

Calories 300

Fat 5g

Fiber 2g

Carbs 12g,

Protein 24g

Creamy Pork and Tomatoes

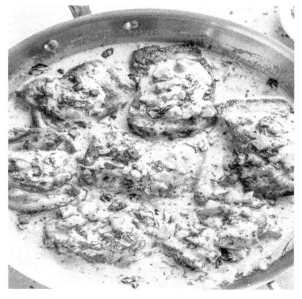

Preparation Time: 10 minutes

Cooking Time: 35 minutes

Servings: 4

Ingredients:

2 pounds pork stew meat, cubed

2 tablespoons avocado oil

1 cup tomatoes, cubed

1 cup coconut cream

1 tablespoon mint, chopped

1 jalapeno pepper, chopped

Pinch of sea salt

Pinch of black pepper

1 tablespoon hot pepper

2 tablespoons lemon juice

Directions:

Warm a pan with the oil over medium heat, add the meat and brown for 5 minutes.

Add the rest of the ingredients, toss, cook over medium heat for 30 minutes more, divide between plates and serve.

Nutrition:

Calories 230

Fat 4g

Fiber 6g

Carbs 9g

Protein 14g

Pork with Balsamic Onion Sauce

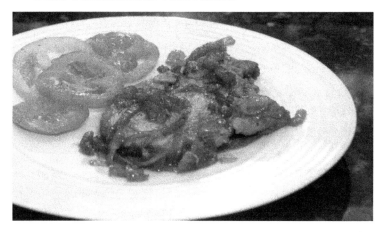

Preparation Time: 10 minutes

Cooking Time: 35 minutes

Servings: 4

Ingredients:

1 yellow onion, chopped

4 scallions, chopped

2 tablespoons avocado oil

1 tablespoon rosemary, chopped

1 tablespoon lemon zest, grated

2 pounds pork roast, sliced

2 tablespoons balsamic vinegar

½ cup vegetable stock

Pinch of sea salt

Pinch black pepper

121

Directions:

Warm a pan with the oil on medium heat, add the onion, and the scallions and sauté for 5 minutes.

Add the rest of the ingredients except the meat, stir, and simmer for 5 minutes.

Add the meat, toss gently, cook over medium heat for 25 minutes, divide between plates and serve.

Nutrition:

Calories 217

Fat 11g

Fiber 1g

Carbs 6g

Protein 14

Buffalo Chicken Lettuce Wraps

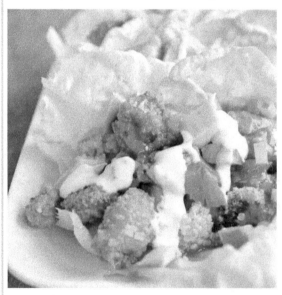

Preparation Time: 15 minutes

Cooking Time: 7 to 8 hours

Servings: 4

Ingredients:

1 tablespoon extra-virgin olive oil

2 pounds boneless, skinless chicken breast

2 cups Vegan Buffalo Dip

1 cup water

8 to 10 romaine lettuce leaves

½ red onion, thinly sliced

1 cup cherry tomatoes, halved

Directions:

Coat the bottom of the slow cooker with olive oil.

Add the chicken, dip, and water, and stir to combine.

Cover the cooker and set to low. Cook for around 7 to 8 hours, or until the internal temperature reaches 165°F on a meat thermometer and the juices run clear.

Shred the chicken using a fork, then mix it into the dip in the slow cooker.

Divide the meat mixture among the lettuce leaves. Top with onion and tomato, and serve.

Nutrition:

Calories: 437

Total Fat: 18g

Total Carbs: 18g

Sugar: 8g

Fiber: 4g

Protein: 49g

Sodium: 993mg

Cilantro-Lime Chicken Drumsticks

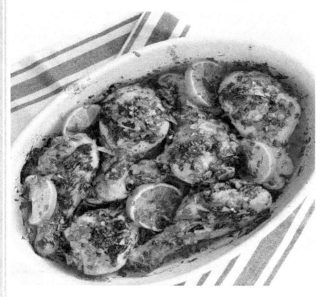

Preparation Time: 15 minutes

Cooking Time: 2 to 3 hours

Servings: 4

Ingredients:

¼ cup fresh cilantro, chopped

3 tablespoons freshly squeezed lime juice

½ teaspoon garlic powder

½ teaspoon sea salt

¼ teaspoon ground cumin

3 pounds chicken drumsticks

Directions:

In a bowl, mix together the cilantro, lime juice, garlic powder, salt, and cumin to form a paste.

Put the drumsticks in the slow cooker. Spread the cilantro paste evenly on each drumstick.

Cover the cooker and set to high. Cook for 2 to 3 hours, or until the internal temperature of the chicken reaches 165°F on a meat thermometer and the juices run clear, and serve (see Tip).

Nutrition:

Calories: 417

Total Fat: 12g

Total Carbs: 1g

Sugar: 1g

Fiber: 1g

Protein: 71g

Sodium: 591mg

Coconut-Curry-Cashew Chicken

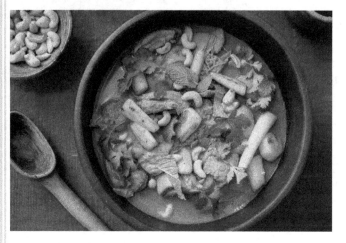

Preparation Time: 15 minutes

Cooking Time: 7 to 8 hours

Servings: 4

Ingredients:

1½ cups Chicken Bone Broth

1 (14-ounce) can full-fat coconut milk

1 teaspoon garlic powder

1 tablespoon red curry paste

1 teaspoon sea salt

½ teaspoon freshly ground black pepper

½ teaspoon coconut sugar

2 pounds boneless, skinless chicken breasts

1½ cup unsalted cashews

½ cup diced white onion

Directions:

In a bowl, combine the broth, coconut milk, garlic powder, red curry paste, salt, pepper, and coconut sugar. Stir well.

Put the chicken, cashews, and onion in the slow cooker. Pour the coconut milk, mixture on top.

Cover the cooker and set to low. Cook for around 7 to 8 hours, or until the internal temperature of the chicken reaches 165°F on a meat thermometer and the juices run clear.

Shred the chicken using a fork, then mix it into the cooking liquid. You can also remove the chicken from the broth and chop it with a knife into bite-size pieces before returning it to the slow cooker. Serve.

Nutrition:

Calories: 714

Total Fat: 43g

Total Carbs: 21g

Sugar: 5g

Fiber: 3g

Protein: 57g

Sodium: 1,606mg

Turkey & Sweet Potato Chili

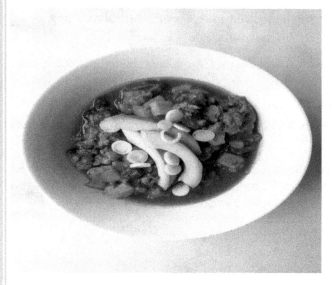

Preparation Time: 15 minutes

Cooking Time: 4 to 6 hours

Servings: 4

Ingredients:

1 tablespoon extra-virgin olive oil

1 pound ground turkey

3 cups sweet potato cubes

1 (28-ounce) can diced tomatoes

1 red bell pepper, diced

1 (4-ounce) can Hatch green chiles

½ medium red onion, diced

2 cups broth of choice

128

1 tablespoon freshly squeezed lime juice

1 tablespoon chili powder

1 teaspoon garlic powder

1 teaspoon cocoa powder

1 teaspoon ground cumin

1 teaspoon sea salt

½ teaspoon ground cinnamon

Pinch cayenne pepper

Directions:

In your slow cooker, combine the olive oil, turkey, sweet potato cubes, tomatoes, bell pepper, chiles, onion, broth, lime juice, chili powder, garlic powder, cocoa powder, cumin, salt, cinnamon, and cayenne. Using a large spoon, break up the turkey into smaller chunks as it combines with the other ingredients.

Cover the cooker and set to low. Cook for 4 to 6 hours.

Stir the chili well, continuing to break up the rest of the turkey, and serve.

Nutrition:

Calories: 380

Total Fat: 12g

Total Carbs: 38g

Sugar: 12g

Fiber: 6g

Protein: 30g

Sodium: 1,268mg

Moroccan Turkey Tagine

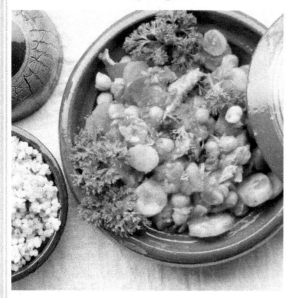

Preparation Time: 15 minutes

Cooking Time: 7 to 8 hours

Servings: 4

Ingredients:

4 cups boneless, skinless turkey breast chunks

1 (14 oz.) can diced tomatoes

1 (14 oz.) can chickpeas, drained

2 large carrots, finely chopped

½ cup dried apricots

½ red onion, chopped

2 tablespoons raw honey

1 tablespoon tomato paste

1 teaspoon garlic powder

1 teaspoon ground turmeric

½ teaspoon sea salt

¼ teaspoon ground ginger

¼ teaspoon ground coriander

¼ teaspoon paprika

½ cup water

2 cups broth of choice

Freshly ground black pepper

Directions:

In your slow cooker, combine the turkey, tomatoes, chickpeas, carrots, apricots, onion, honey, tomato paste, garlic powder, turmeric, salt, ginger, coriander, paprika, water, and broth, and season with pepper. Gently stir to blend the ingredients.

Cover the cooker and set to low. Cook for 7 to 8 hours and serve.

Nutrition:

Calories: 428

Total Fat: 5g

Total Carbs: 46g

Sugar: 25g

Fiber: 8g

Protein: 49g

Sodium: 983mg

Wasabi Salmon Burgers

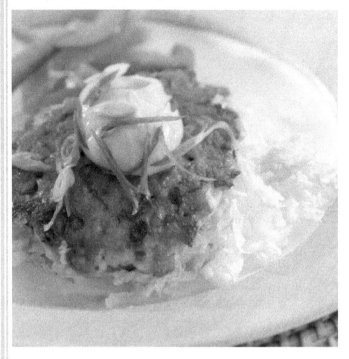

Preparation Time: 5 minutes

Cooking Time: 10 minutes

Servings: 1

Ingredients:

1/2 tsp. Honey

2 tbsp. Reduce-salt soy sauce

1 tsp. Wasabi powder

1 Beaten free-range egg

2 can Wild Salmon, drained

132

2 Scallion, chopped

2 tbsp. Coconut Oil

1 tbsp. Fresh ginger, minced

Directions:

Combine the salmon, egg, ginger, scallions, and 1 tbsp oil in a bowl, mixing well with your hands to form 4 patties.

In a separate bowl, add the wasabi powder and soy sauce with the honey and whisk until blended.

Heat 1 tbsp oil over medium heat in a skillet and cook the patties for 4 minutes each side until firm and browned.

Glaze the top of each patty with the wasabi mixture and cook for another 15 seconds before you serve.

Serve with your favorite side salad or vegetables for a healthy treat.

Nutrition:

Calories: 591 kcal

Protein: 63.52 g

Fat: 34.3 g

Carbohydrates: 3.83 g

Citrus & Herb Sardines

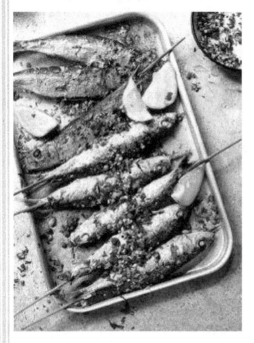

Preparation Time: 5 minutes

Cooking Time: 15 minutes

Servings: 2

Ingredients:

10 Sardines, scaled and clean

2 Whole Lemon zest

Handful-Flat leafy parsley, chopped

2 Garlic cloves, finely chopped

1/2 cup Black Olives (pitted and halves)

3 tbsp. Olive oil

1 can Tomato, chopped, (optional)

1/2 can Chickpeas or Butterbeans, drained and rinsed

8 Cherry Tomatoes, halved (optional)

Pinch of Black Pepper

Directions:

In a bowl, add the lemon zest to the chopped parsley (save a pinch for garnishing) and half of the chopped garlic, ready for later.

Put a very large skillet on the hob and heat on high.

Now add the oil and once very hot, lay the sardines flat on the pan.

Sauté for 3 minutes until golden underneath and turn over to fry for another 3 minutes. Place onto a plate to rest.

Sauté the remaining garlic (add another splash of oil if you need to) for 1 min until softened. Pour in the tin of chopped tomatoes, mix and let simmer for 4-5 minutes.

If you're avoiding tomatoes, just avoid this step and go straight to chickpeas.

Tip in the chickpeas or butter beans and fresh tomatoes and stir until heated through.

Here's when you add the sardines into the lemon and parsley dressing prepared earlier and add to the pan, cooking for a further 3-4 minutes.

Once heated through, serve with a pinch of parsley and remaining lemon zest to garnish.

Nutrition:

Calories: 493 kcal

Protein: 24.16 g

Fat: 35.67 g

Carbohydrates: 20.92 g

Super Sesame Chicken Noodles

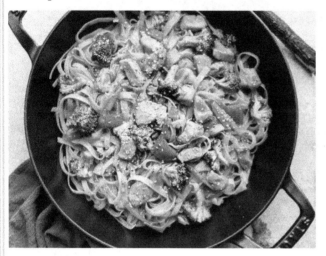

Preparation Time: 10 minutes

Cooking Time: 10 minutes

Servings: 2

Ingredients:

2 Free-range skinless chicken breasts, chopped

1 cup Rice/Buckwheat noodles such as Japanese Udon

1 Carrot, chopped

1/2 orange juiced

1 tsp. Sesame Seed

2 tsp. Coconut Oil

1 Thumb size piece of ginger, minced

1/2 cup Sugar snap peas

Directions:

Warm 1 tsp oil on medium heat in a skillet.

Sauté the chopped chicken breast for about 10-15 minutes or until cooked through.

While cooking the chicken, place the noodles, carrots, and peas in a pot of boiling water for about 5 minutes. Drain.

In a bowl, mix together the ginger, sesame seeds, 1 tsp oil, and orange juice to make your dressing.

Once the chicken is cooked and noodles are cooked and drained, add the chicken, noodles, carrots, and peas to the dressing and toss.

Serve warm or chilled.

Nutrition:

Calories: 168 kcal

Protein: 5.31 g

Fat: 8.66 g

Carbohydrates: 19.34 g

Lebanese Chicken Kebabs and Hummus

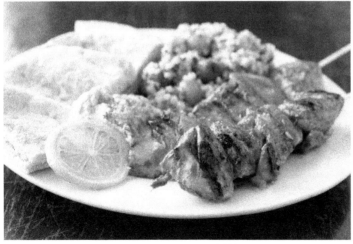

Preparation Time: 10 minutes + 1 hour marinate

Cooking Time: 35 minutes

Servings: 4

Ingredients:

For the Chicken:

1 cup Lemon Juice

8 Garlic cloves, minced

1 tbsp. Thyme, finely chopped

1 tbsp. Paprika

2 tsp. ground cumin

1 tsp. Cayenne pepper

4 Free-range skinless chicken breasts, cubed

4 Metal kebabs skewers

Lemon wedges to garnish

For the Hummus:

1 can Chickpeas/ 1 cup dried (soaked overnight)

2 tbsp. Tahini paste

1 Lemon juice

1 tsp. Turmeric

1 tsp. Black pepper

2 tbsp. Olive oil

Directions:

Whisk the lemon juice, garlic, thyme, paprika, cumin, and cayenne pepper in a bowl.

Skewer the chicken cubes using kebab sticks (metal).

Baste the chicken per side with the marinade, covering for as long as possible in the fridge (the lemon juice will tenderize the meat and means it will be more suitable for the anti-inflammatory diet).

When ready to cook, set the oven to 400°F/200 °C/Gas Mark 6 and bake for 20-25 minutes or until chicken is thoroughly cooked through.

Prepare the hummus by putting the ingredients to a blender and whizzing up until smooth. If it is a little thick and chunky, add a little water to loosen the mix.

Serve the chicken kebabs, garnished with the lemon wedges and the hummus on the side.

Nutrition:

Calories: 576 kcal

Protein: 61.66 g

Fat: 18.55 g

Carbohydrates: 42.07 g

Manhattan-Style Salmon Chowder

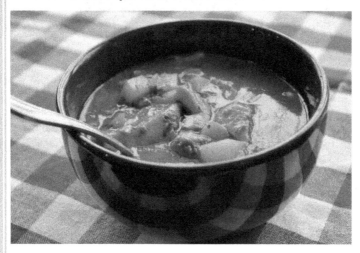

Preparation Time: 10 minutes

Cooking Time: 15 minutes

Servings: 4

Ingredients:

¼ cup Extra Virgin Olive Oil

1 Red Bell Pepper, Chopped

1 Pound Skinless Salmon. Pin Bones removed, chopped into ½ inch

2 (28 oz.) Cans Crushed Tomatoes, 1 Drained, 1 undrained

6 cups No salt added chicken broth

2 cups diced (1/2 inch) Sweet Potato

1 tsp. Onion Powder

½ tsp. Sea Salt

¼ tsp. Freshly Ground Black Pepper

Directions:

Add the red bell pepper and salmon. Cook for at least 5 minutes, occasionally stirring, until the fish is opaque and the bell pepper is soft.

Stir in the tomatoes, chicken broth, sweet potatoes, onion powder, salt, and pepper. Place to a simmer then lower the heat to medium. Cook for at least 10 minutes, occasionally stirring, until the sweet potatoes are soft.

Nutrition:

Calories: 570

Total Fat: 42

Total Carbs: 55g

Sugar: 24g

Fiber: 16g

Protein: 41g

Sodium: 1,249mg

Roasted Salmon and Asparagus

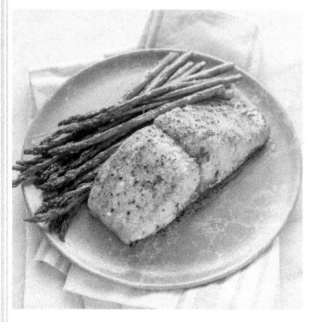

Preparation Time: 5 minutes

Cooking Time: 15 minutes

Servings: 4

Ingredients:

1 pound Asparagus Spears, trimmed

2 tbsp. Extra Virgin Olive Oil

1 tsp. Sea Salt, divide

1½ pound Salmon, cut into 4 fillets

⅛ tsp. freshly ground cracked black pepper

142

1 Lemon, zest, and slice

Directions:

Preheat the oven to 425°F.

Stir the asparagus with the olive oil then put ½ teaspoon of the salt. Place in a single layer in the bottom of a roasting pan.

Season the salmon with the pepper and the remaining ½ teaspoon of salt. Put skin-side down on top of the asparagus.

Sprinkle the salmon and asparagus with the lemon zest and place the lemon slices over the fish.

Roast at the oven for at least 12 to 15 minutes until the flesh is opaque.

Nutrition:

Calories: 308

Total Fat: 18g

Total Carbs: 5g

Sugar: 2g

Fiber: 2g

Protein: 36g

Sodium: 545mg

Citrus Salmon on a Bed of Greens

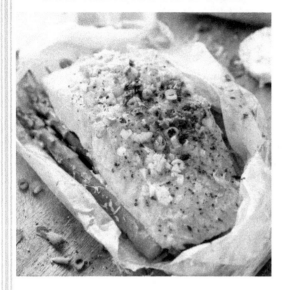

Preparation Time: 10 minutes

Cooking Time: 19 minutes

Servings: 4

Ingredients:

¼ cup Extra Virgin Olive Oil, divided

1½ pound Salmon

1 tsp. Sea Salt, divided

½ tsp. Freshly ground black pepper, divided

1 Lemon Zest

6 cups Swiss Chard, stemmed and chopped

3 Garlic cloves, chopped

2 Lemon Juice

Directions:

In a huge nonstick skillet at medium-high heat, heat 2 tablespoons of the olive oil until it shimmers.

Season the salmon with ½ teaspoon of the salt, ¼ teaspoon of the pepper, and the lemon zest. Put the salmon to the skillet, skin-side up, and cook for about 7 minutes until the flesh is opaque. Flip the salmon and cook for at least 3 to 4 minutes to crisp the skin. Set aside on a plate, cover using aluminum foil.

Put back the skillet to the heat, add the remaining 2 tablespoons of olive oil, and heat it until it shimmers.

Add the Swiss chard. Cook for about 7 minutes, occasionally stirring, until soft.

Add the garlic. Cook for 30 seconds, stirring constantly.

Sprinkle in the lemon juice, the remaining ½ teaspoon of salt, and the remaining ¼ teaspoon of pepper. Cook for 2 minutes.

Serve the salmon on the Swiss chard.

Nutrition:

Calories: 363

Total Fat: 25

Total Carbs: 3g

Sugar: 1g

Fiber: 1g

Protein: 34g

Sodium: 662mg

Orange and Maple-Glazed Salmon

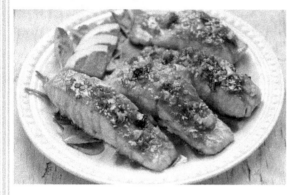

Preparation Time: 15 minutes

Cooking Time: 15 minutes

Servings: 4

Ingredients:

2 Orange Juice

1 Orange Zest

¼ cup Pure maple syrup

2 tbsp. Low Sodium Soy Sauce

1 tsp. Garlic Powder

4 4-6 oz. Salmon Fillet, Pin bones removed

Directions:

Preheat the oven to 400°F.

In a small, shallow dish, whisk the orange juice and zest, maple syrup, soy sauce, and garlic powder.

Put the salmon pieces, flesh-side down, into the dish. Let it marinate for 10 minutes.

Transfer the salmon, skin-side up, to a rimmed baking sheet and bake for about 15 minutes until the flesh is opaque.

Nutrition:

Calories: 297

Total Fat: 11

Total Carbs: 18g

Sugar: 15g

Fiber: 1g

Protein: 34g

Sodium: 528mg

Dinner

Lemony Mussels

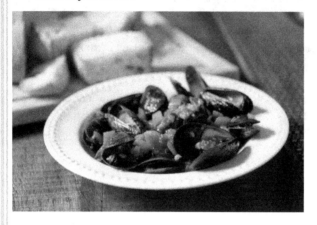

Preparation Time: 5 minutes

Cooking Time: 5 minutes

Servings: 4

Ingredients:

1 tbsp. extra virgin extra virgin olive oil

2 minced garlic cloves

2 lbs. scrubbed mussels

Juice of one lemon

Directions:

Put some water in a pot, add mussels, bring with a boil over medium heat, cook for 5 minutes, discard unopened mussels and transfer them with a bowl.

In another bowl, mix the oil with garlic and freshly squeezed lemon juice, whisk well, and add over the mussels, toss and serve.

Enjoy!

Nutrition:

Calories: 140

Fat: 4 g

Carbs: 8 g

Protein: 8 g

Sugars: 4g

Sodium: 600 mg

Hot Tuna Steak

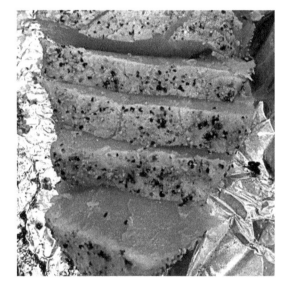

Preparation Time: 10 minutes

Cooking Time: 25 minutes

Servings: 6

Ingredients:

2 tbsps. Fresh lemon juice

Pepper.

Roasted orange garlic mayonnaise

¼ c. whole black peppercorns

6 sliced tuna steaks

2 tbsps. Extra-virgin olive oil

Salt

Directions:

Bring the tuna in a bowl to fit. Put the oil, lemon juice, salt, and pepper. Turn the tuna to coat well in the marinade.

Rest for at least 15 to 20 minutes, turning once.

Put the peppercorns in a double thickness of plastic bags. Tap the peppercorns with a heavy saucepan or small mallet to crush them coarsely. Put on a large plate.

Once ready to cook the tuna, dip the edges into the crushed peppercorns. Heat a nonstick skillet over medium heat. Sear the tuna steaks, in batches if necessary, for 4 minutes per side for medium-rare fish, adding 2 to 3 tablespoons of the marinade to the skillet if necessary, to prevent sticking.

Serve dolloped with roasted orange garlic mayonnaise

Nutrition:

Calories: 124

Fat: 0.4 g

Carbs: 0.6 g

Protein: 28 g

Sugars: 0 g

Sodium: 77 mg

Marinated Fish Steaks

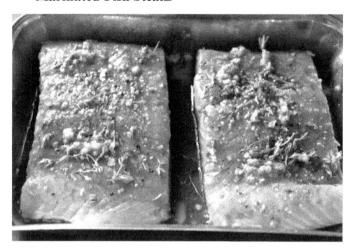

Preparation Time: 10 minutes

Cooking Time: 15 minutes

Servings: 4

Ingredients:

4 lime wedges

2 tbsps. Lime juice

2 minced garlic cloves

2 tsp. Olive oil

1 tbsp. snipped fresh oregano

1 lb. fresh swordfish

1 tsp. lemon-pepper seasoning

Directions:

Rinse fish steaks; pat dry using paper towels. Cut into four serving-size pieces, if necessary.

151

In a shallow dish, put and combine lime juice, oregano, oil, lemon-pepper seasoning, and garlic. Add fish; turn to coat with marinade.

Broil 4 inches from the heat for at least 8 to 12 minutes or until fish starts to flake when tested with a fork, turning once and brushing with reserved marinade halfway through cooking.

Take off any remaining marinade.

Before serving, squeeze the lime juice on each steak.

Nutrition:

Calories: 240

 Fat: 6 g

Carbs: 19 g

Protein: 12 g

Sugars: 3.27 g

Sodium: 325 mg

Baked Tomato Hake

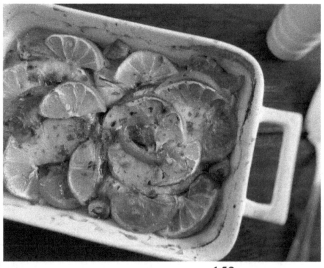

152

Preparation Time: 10 minutes

Cooking Time: 20-25 minutes

Servings: 4

Ingredients:

½ c. tomato sauce

1 tbsp. olive oil

Parsley

2 sliced tomatoes

½ c. grated cheese

4 lbs. de-boned and sliced hake fish

Salt.

Directions:

Preheat the oven to 400 0F.

Season the fish with salt.

In a skillet or saucepan, stir-fry the fish in the olive oil until half-done.

Take four foil papers to cover the fish.

Shape the foil to resemble containers; add the tomato sauce into each foil container.

Add the fish, tomato slices, and top with grated cheese.

Bake until you get a golden crust, for approximately 20-25 minutes.

Open the packs and top with parsley.

Nutrition:

Calories: 265

Fat: 15 g

Carbs: 18 g

Protein: 22 g

Sugars: 0.5 g

Sodium: 94.6 mg

Cheesy Tuna Pasta

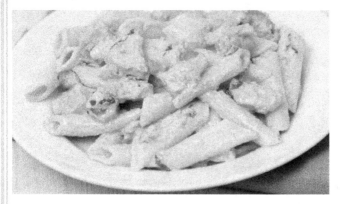

Preparation Time: 10 minutes

Cooking Time: 20 minutes

Servings: 2-4

Ingredients:

2 c. arugula

¼ c. chopped green onions

1 tbs. red vinegar

5 oz. drained canned tuna

¼ tsp. black pepper

2 oz. cooked whole-wheat pasta

1 tbsp. olive oil

1 tbsp. grated low-fat parmesan

Directions:

Cook the pasta in unsalted water until ready. Drain and set aside.

In a large-sized bowl, thoroughly mix the tuna, green onions, vinegar, oil, arugula, pasta, and black pepper.

Toss well and top with the cheese.

Serve and enjoy.

Nutrition:

Calories: 566.3

Fat: 42.4 g

Carbs: 18.6 g

Protein: 29.8 g

Sugars: 0.4 g

Sodium: 688.6 mg

Salmon and Roasted Peppers

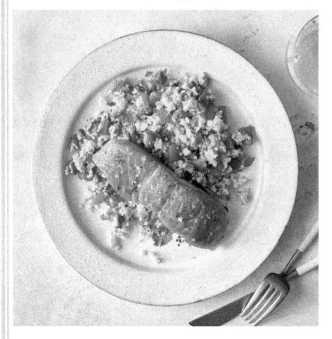

Preparation Time: 5 minutes

Cooking Time: 25 minutes

Servings: 4

Ingredients:

1 cup red peppers, cut into strips

4 salmon fillets, boneless

¼ cup chicken stock

2 tablespoons olive oil

1 yellow onion, chopped

1 tablespoon cilantro, chopped

Pinch of sea salt

Pinch black pepper

Directions:

Warm a pan with the oil on medium-high heat; add the onion and sauté for 5 minutes.

Put the fish and cook for at least 5 minutes on each side.

Add the rest of the ingredients, introduce the pan in the oven, and cook at 390 degrees F for 10 minutes.

Divide the mix between plates and serve.

Nutrition:

Calories 265

Fat 7g

Fiber 5g

Carbs 15g

Protein 16g

Golden Chickpea And Vegetable Soup

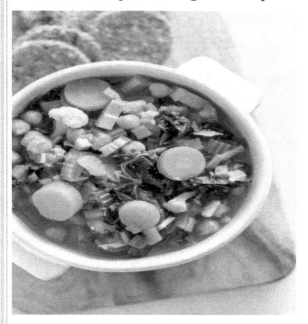

Preparation Time: 15 minutes

Cooking Time: 20 minutes

Servings: 6

Ingredients:

1 tbsp. Grated ginger

1 cup diced carrots

2 tsp. Coconut oil

2 tbsp. Curry powder

2 cups Cauliflower florets

2 cloves minced garlic

1 cup cooked chickpeas

1 ½ cup Diced celery

1 ½ cup Sliced leeks

4 cups Bone broth

2 tbsp. Minced organic parsley

1 cup Torn curly kale leaves

Directions:

Warm the coconut oil in a pot and add the garlic and ginger. Sauté for a minute before adding the turmeric and curry powder and sautéing for another minute.

Throw in celery, leeks, carrots, and cauliflower, constantly stirring for about a minute.

Add the bone broth and chickpeas. Cover the pot and leave to boil. Lower the heat and let it simmer for at least 15 minutes.

Turn off heat and add parsley and kale, leaving the heat to cook the leaves.

Sprinkle salt and pepper.

Serve.

Nutrition:

Calories: 142 kcal

Protein: 8.64 g

Fat: 4.79 g

Carbohydrates: 17.57 g

Anti-inflammatory Spring Pea Soup

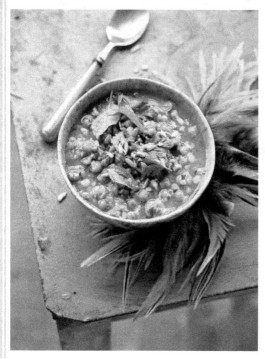

Preparation Time: 5 minutes

Cooking Time: 15 minutes

Servings: 6

Ingredients:

2 tbsp. Coconut oil

700 g. Fresh peas

1 medium Chopped onion

Chopped mint leaves

1 liter Vegetable stock

Chopped flat-leaf parsley

Fresh lemon juice

½ tsp. ground cumin

2 tsp. Celtic sea salt

Toasted sunflower seeds

Grated nutmeg

½ tsp. Black pepper powder

Directions:

Warm the coconut oil in a pan set over medium heat.

Stir in onions and stir fry for about 5 minutes.

Put in the stock and raise the heat. Throw in fresh peas and cook for 5 minutes. If you're using frozen peas, it should take half the time.

Pour in the lemon juice, salt, pepper, herbs, and spices. Stirring constantly

Turn off the heat and let it cool before running it through a food processor to whatever consistency you like.

Serve with sunflower seed sprinkles and mint or parsley leaves.

Enjoy!

Nutrition:

Calories: 115 kcal

Protein: 5 g

Fat: 5.91 g

Carbohydrates: 11.8 g

Roasted Butternut Squash Apple Soup

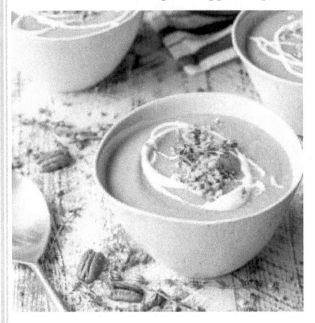

Preparation Time: 10 minutes

Cooking Time: 40 minutes

Servings: 4

Ingredients:

2 red, sweet apples

3 cups low-sodium chicken/vegetable stock

1 butternut squash

1/4 teaspoon nutmeg

4 tablespoons olive oil

1 small onion

1/4 teaspoon ginger

1 celery rib

1/4 teaspoon cinnamon

1 cup water

Salt & pepper to taste

Directions:

Preheat the oven to 400°F.

Place diced apple on a one-sheet pan & place the diced butternut squash on the second sheet pan.

Allow season to squash olive oil & add pepper & salt. Stir get everything mix well. Add apple with one tablespoon olive oil & stir to coat.

Apple & Roast squash for 25-30 minutes, until browned.

Heat olive oil (remaining 1 1/2 tablespoons) in a large stockpot.

Sauté celery & onion for 6-8 minutes, until tender. Add Pepper & salt to taste.

Add vegetable or chicken stock & water & bring to a simmer.

Once the apple & squash are roasted, add them to the pot. Add cinnamon, nutmeg & ginger.

Now blend the soup until smooth. Season pepper & salt to taste.

Serve with desired toppings.

Nutrition:

Calories: 251 kcal

Protein: 4.06 g

Fat: 15.93 g

Carbohydrates: 25.14 g

Herbed Rockfish

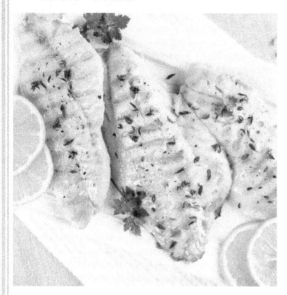

Preparation Time: 10 minutes

Cooking Time: 20 minutes

Servings: 8

Ingredients:

1 1/2 pounds rockfish fillets

2 egg whites

1 1/2 tablespoons nonfat milk

1/2 tablespoons canola oil

1 cup nonfat plain yogurt

1 tablespoon lemon juice

1 tablespoon oregano

1 tablespoon fresh parsley, chopped

164

1 tablespoon pimento, minced

1 teaspoon garlic, minced

1 teaspoon ground black pepper

6 slices wheat bread, toasted

1/4 cup flaxseed, ground fresh

1/4 cup extra virgin olive oil

1 pint cherry tomatoes, chopped

2 fresh lemons, wedges

Directions:

Clean rockfish fillets in cold water, remove the skin and remove any bones — Pat dry with paper towels. In a medium-size bowl, combine egg whites, nonfat milk, yogurt, canola oil, and lemon juice — place in a pie pan.

Put the next 8 ingredients (oregano-flaxseed) in a food processor until finely ground — place in a separate dish.

Heat the olive oil in a pan. First, soak the fillets in the spice mixture, succeeded by the yogurt blend, and then once again in the spice mixture, compressing the crumbs gently into the fish for the final layer.

Place the fillets in hot olive oil. When the underneath begins to brown, flip the fillets over, and reduce heat — Cook for a further 15 to 20 minutes.

Complete with tomatoes and lemon wedges.

Nutrition:

Calories: 178 kcal

Protein: 19.62 g

Fat: 8.96 g

Carbohydrates: 4.73 g

Salmon Sushi

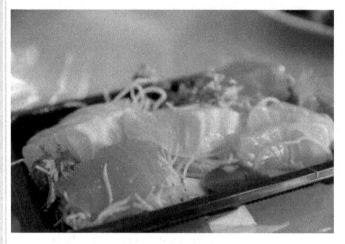

Preparation Time: 30 minutes

Cooking Time: 20 minutes

Servings: 26

Ingredients:

1 1/2 cups water

1 cup of sushi rice

1/2 tablespoons rice vinegar

1/2 teaspoons sugar

1 teaspoon salt

4 ounces smoked salmon

4 nori seaweed sheets

Optional: low-sodium soy sauce or wasabi paste.

Directions:

166

Using a pot with a lid, bring water to a boil. Combine rice, cover, and lessen the temperature.

Simmer 18 to 20 minutes, turn off the heat, and leave the rice to cool for 10 minutes. Place the rice in a bowl and dampen with vinegar, salt, and sugar. Blend with a wooden spoon, and allow the rice to stand. Chop smoked salmon into strips.

Make each sushi roll as follows:

Place 1 seaweed layer on a clean, dry surface.

Place 1/2 cup cooked rice over the seaweed, and delicately spread evenly over the sheet. Lay the strips of salmon in a perpendicular line in the center of the rice.

Delicately roll so as not to rip the seaweed, starting at the left edge, and ending just before the right edge — Tuck rice in at the sides of the roll.

Run a damp finger along the exhibited edge of the seaweed, and conclude rolling, pressing down to seal the border to the roll.

Slice into pieces using a cutting knife.

Nutrition:

Calories: 25 kcal

Protein: 1.78 g

Fat: 1.49 g

Carbohydrates: 2.33 g

Apricot Chicken Wings

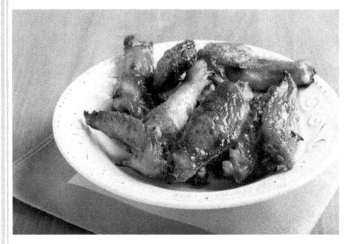

Preparation Time: 15 minutes

Cooking Time: 45-60 minutes

Servings: 3-4

Ingredients:

1 medium jar apricot preserve

1 package Lipton onion dry soup mix

1 medium bottle Russian dressing

2 lbs. chicken wings

Directions:

Preheat the oven to 350∘F.

Rinse and pat dry the chicken wings.

Bring the chicken wings on a baking pan, single layer.

Bake for 45 – 60 minutes, turning halfway.

In a medium bowl, combine the Lipton soup mix, apricot preserve, and Russian dressing.

Once the wings are cooked, toss with the sauce, until the pieces are coated.

Serve immediately with a side dish.

Nutrition:

Calories: 162

Fat:17 g

Carbs:76 g

Protein:13 g

Sugars:24 g

Sodium:700 mg

Honey Chicken Tagine

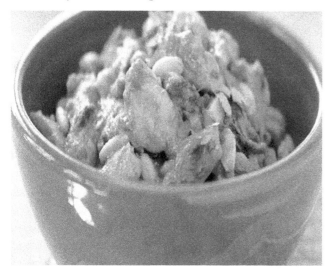

Preparation Time: 60 minutes

Cooking Time: 25 minutes

Servings: 12

Ingredients:

1 tbsp. extra virgin olive oil

1 tsp. ground coriander

1 tbsp. Minced fresh ginger

½ tsp. ground pepper

2 thinly sliced onions

12-oz. seeded and roughly chopped kumquats

14-oz. vegetable broth

1/8 tsp. Ground cloves

½ tsp. salt

1 ½ tbsps. honey

1 tsp. ground cumin

2 lbs. boneless, skinless chicken thighs

4 slivered garlic cloves

15-oz rinsed chickpeas

¾ tsp. ground cinnamon

Directions:

Preheat the oven to about 3750F.

Put a heatproof casserole on medium heat and heat the oil.

Add onions to sauté for 4 minutes

Add garlic and ginger to sauté for 1 minute

Add coriander, cumin, cloves, salt, pepper, and cloves seasonings. Sauté for a minute.

Add kumquats, broth, chickpeas, and honey, then bring to a boil before turning off the heat.

Set the casserole in the oven while covered. Bake for 15 minutes as you stir at a 15-minute interval.

Serve and enjoy

Nutrition:

Calories: 586 kcal

Protein: 15.5 g

Fat: 40.82 g

Carbohydrates: 43.56 g

Roasted Chicken

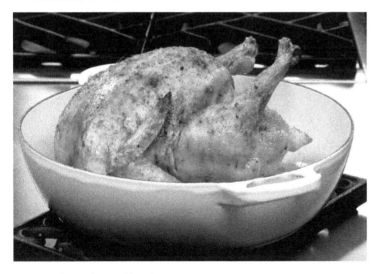

Preparation Time: 60 minutes

Cooking Time: 60 minutes

171

Servings: 8

Ingredients:

½ tsp. thyme

3 lbs. whole chicken

1 bay leaf

3 garlic cloves

4 tbsps. Coarsely chopped orange peel

½ tsp. Black pepper

½ tbsp. salt

Directions:

Put the chicken under room temperature for about 1 hour.

Using paper towels, pat dry the inside and outside of the chicken.

Preheat the oven to 4500F as soon as you start preparing the chicken seasoning.

Combine thyme, salt, and pepper in a small bowl.

Wipe inside the using 1/3 of the seasoning. Inside the chicken, put the garlic, citrus peel, and bay leaf.

Tuck the tips of the wing and tie the legs together. Spread the rest of the seasoning all over the chicken and put on a roasting pan.

Put in the oven to bake for 60 minutes at 1600F.

Set aside to rest for 15 minutes.

Cut up the roasted chicken and serve.

Enjoy.

Nutrition:

Calories: 201 kcal

Protein: 35.48 g

Fat: 5.36 g

Carbohydrates: 0.5 g

Chicken in Pita Bread

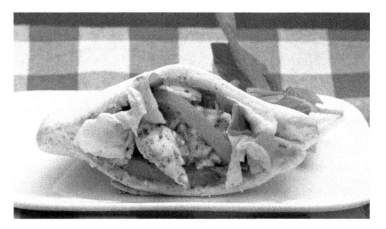

Preparation Time: 10 minutes

Cooking Time: 10 minutes

Servings: 4

Ingredients:

1 tbsp. Greek seasoning blend

Two lightly beaten large egg whites

½ c. chopped green onions

½ c. diced tomato

2 c. shredded lettuce

4 pieces of 6-inch halved pitas

2 tsp. Divided grated lemon rind

173

½ c. plain low-fat yogurt

1 tbsp. olive oil

1 ½ tsps. chopped fresh oregano

1 lb. Ground chicken

½ tsp. coarsely ground black pepper

Directions:

Combine egg whites, Greek seasoning, a tablespoon lemon rind, green onions, and black pepper. Separate into 8 parts and mold each into ¼ inch thick patty.

Adjust your heat to medium-high. Set a non-stick skillet in place and fry patties until browned.

Lower the heat to medium. Then, cover the skillet to cook for 4 more minutes.

Set up a small bowl and combine yogurt, oregano, and a tablespoon of lemon rind.

Spread the mixture on the pita and add ¼ cup lettuce and a tablespoon of tomato.

Nutrition:

Calories: 421 kcal

Protein: 29.72 g

Fat: 23.37 g

Carbohydrates: 23.26 g

Orange Chicken Legs

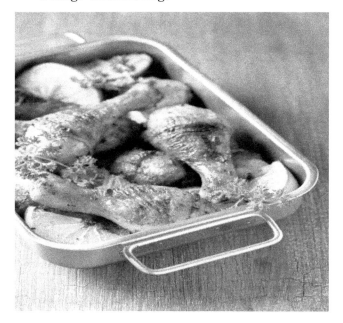

Preparation Time: 10 minutes

Cooking Time: 8 hours

Servings: 4

Ingredients:

Zest of 1 orange

Juice of 1 orange

¼ cup red vinegar

A pinch of salt and black pepper

4 chicken legs

5 garlic cloves, minced

1 red onion, cut into wedges

175

7 ounces canned peaches, halved

½ cup chopped parsley

Directions:

In a slow cooker, mix the orange zest with the orange juice, vinegar, salt, pepper, garlic, onion, peaches, and parsley. Add the chicken, toss, cover, and cook on Low for 8 hours. Divide between plates and serve.

Enjoy!

Nutrition:

Calories:251

Fat: 4g

Fiber: 8g

Carbs: 14g

Protein: 8g

Spicy Herb Catfish

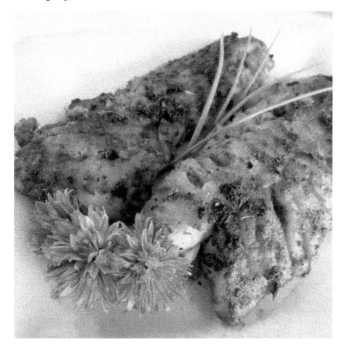

Preparation Time: 10 minutes

Cooking Time: 25 minutes

Servings: 4

Ingredients:

For the spice mixture:

1/4 cup coriander seeds

1/2 teaspoons cumin seeds

1/2 tablespoon ground red pepper

1/2 teaspoon crushed cardamom

1 tablespoon raw sugar

1 tablespoon kosher salt

1 teaspoon ground black pepper

Four 6-ounce catfish fillets

1/2 cup flaxseed, freshly ground

Canola oil spray

For the garnish:

Several sprigs of fresh cilantro 1 medium tomato and

  1 lemon quartered

Directions:

Preheat oven to 350°F. Place the spice blend ingredients into a mixing bowl, and combine well. Place the mixture inside a pie pan.

Clean the catfish fillets and pat dry. Put ground flaxseed into an alternate pie pan. Dredge fillets in the spice mixture first, followed by flaxseed. Spray the baking sheet with canola oil and place fillets on a baking sheet and cook for 18 minutes. Boil the stock juices for an additional 6 minutes. Pour the juices over the fillets and serve decorated with cilantro, a portion of tomato, and a lemon quarter.

Nutrition:

Calories: 208 kcal

Protein: 13.5 g

Fat: 12.65 g

Carbohydrates: 13.66 g

Beef with Zucchini Noodles

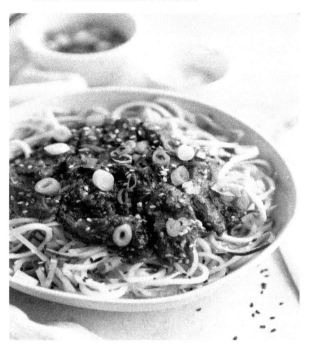

Preparation Time: 15 minutes

Cooking Time: 9 minutes

Servings: 4

Ingredients:

1 teaspoon fresh ginger, grated

2 medium garlic cloves, minced

¼ cup coconut aminos

2 tablespoons fresh lime juice

1½ pound NY strip steak, trimmed and sliced thinly

2 medium zucchinis, spiralized with Blade C

Salt, to taste

3 tablespoons essential olive oil

2 medium scallions, sliced

1 teaspoon red pepper flakes, crushed

2 tablespoons fresh cilantro, chopped

Directions:

In a big bowl, mix together ginger, garlic, coconut aminos, and lime juice.

Add beef and coat with marinade generously.

Refrigerate to marinate for approximately 10 minutes.

Place zucchini noodles over a large paper towel and sprinkle with salt.

Keep aside for around 10 minutes.

In a big skillet, heat oil on medium-high heat.

Add scallion and red pepper flakes and sauté for about 1 minute.

Add beef with marinade and stir fry for around 3-4 minutes or till browned.

Add zucchini and cook for approximately 3-4 minutes.

Serve hot with all the topping of cilantro.

Nutrition:

Calories: 434

 Fat: 17g

Carbohydrates: 23g

 Fiber: 12g

Protein: 29g

Beef with Asparagus & Bell Pepper

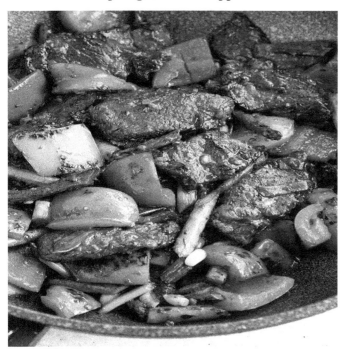

Preparation Time: 15 minutes

Cooking Time: 13 minutes

Servings: 4-5

Ingredients:

4 garlic cloves, minced

3 tablespoons coconut aminos

1/8 teaspoon red pepper flakes, crushed

1/8 teaspoon ground ginger

Freshly ground black pepper, to taste

181

1 bunch asparagus, trimmed and halved

2 tablespoons olive oil, divided

1-pound flank steak, trimmed and sliced thinly

1 red bell pepper, seeded and sliced

3 tablespoons water

2 teaspoons arrowroot powder

Directions:

In a bowl, mix together garlic, coconut aminos, red pepper flakes, crushed, ground ginger, and black pepper. Keep aside.

In a pan of boiling water, cook asparagus for about 2 minutes.

Drain and rinse under cold water.

In a substantial skillet, heat 1 tablespoon of oil on medium-high heat.

Add beef and stir fry for around 3-4 minutes.

With a slotted spoon, transfer the beef in a bowl.

In a similar skillet, heat remaining oil on medium heat.

Add asparagus and bell pepper and stir fry for approximately 2-3 minutes.

Meanwhile, in the bowl, mix together water and arrowroot powder.

Stir in beef, garlic mixture, and arrowroot mixture, and cook for around 3-4 minutes or till desired thickness.

Nutrition:

Calories: 399

Fat: 17g

Carbohydrates: 27g

 Fiber: 8g

Protein: 35g

Spiced Ground Beef

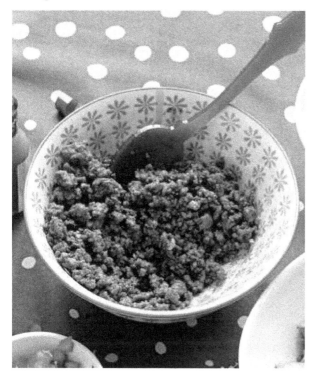

Preparation Time: 10 minutes

Cooking Time: 22 minutes

Servings: 5

Ingredients:

2 tablespoons coconut oil

2 whole cloves

2 whole cardamoms

1 (2-inch piece cinnamon stick

183

2 bay leaves

1 teaspoon cumin seeds

2 onions, chopped

Salt, to taste

½ tablespoon garlic paste

½ tablespoon fresh ginger paste

1-pound lean ground beef

1½ teaspoons fennel seeds powder

1 teaspoon ground cumin

1½ teaspoons red chili powder

1/8 teaspoon ground turmeric

Freshly ground black pepper, to taste

1 cup coconut milk

¼ cup water

¼ cup fresh cilantro, chopped

Directions:

In a sizable pan, heat oil on medium heat.

Add cloves, cardamoms, cinnamon stick, bay leaves, and cumin seeds and sauté for about 20-a few seconds.

Add onion and 2 pinches of salt and sauté for about 3-4 minutes.

Add garlic-ginger paste and sauté for about 2 minutes.

Add beef and cook for about 4-5 minutes, entering pieces using the spoon.

Cover and cook approximately 5 minutes.

Stir in spices and cook, stirring for approximately 2-2½ minutes.

Stir in coconut milk and water and cook for about 7-8 minutes.

Season with salt and take away from heat.

Serve hot using the garnishing of cilantro.

Nutrition:

Calories: 444

Fat: 15g

Carbohydrates: 29g

Fiber: 11g

Protein: 39g

Ground Beef with Cabbage

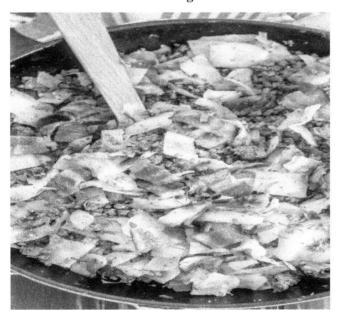

Preparation Time: 10 minutes

Cooking Time: 15 minutes

Servings: 6

Ingredients:

1 tbsp. olive oil

1 onion, sliced thinly

2 teaspoons fresh ginger, minced

4 garlic cloves, minced

1-pound lean ground beef

1½ tablespoons fish sauce

2 tablespoons fresh lime juice

1 small head purple cabbage, shredded

2 tablespoons peanut butter

½ cup fresh cilantro, chopped

Directions:

In a huge skillet, warm oil on medium heat.

Add onion, ginger, and garlic and sauté for about 4-5 minutes.

Add beef and cook for approximately 7-8 minutes, getting into pieces using the spoon.

Drain off the extra liquid in the skillet.

Stir in fish sauce and lime juice and cook for approximately 1 minute.

Add cabbage and cook approximately 4-5 minutes or till desired doneness.

Stir in peanut butter and cilantro and cook for about 1 minute.

Serve hot.

Nutrition:

Calories: 402

Fat: 13g

Carbohydrates: 21g

Fiber: 10g

Protein: 33g

Roasted Root Vegetables

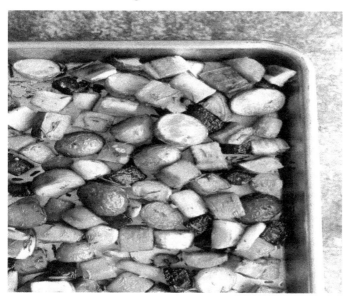

Preparation Time: 10 minutes

Cooking Time: 1 hour and 30 minutes

Servings: 6

Ingredients:

2 tbsp. olive oil

187

1 head garlic, cloves separated and peeled

1 large turnip, peeled and cut into ½-inch pieces

1 medium-sized red onion, cut into ½-inch pieces

1 ½ lb. beets, trimmed but not peeled, scrubbed and cut into ½-inch pieces

1 ½ lb. Yukon gold potatoes, unpeeled, cut into ½-inch pieces

2 ½ lbs. butternut squash, peeled, seeded, cut into ½-inch pieces

Directions:

Grease 2 rimmed and large baking sheets. Preheat oven to 425oF.

In a huge bowl, mix all ingredients thoroughly.

Into the two baking sheets, evenly divide the root vegetables, spread in one layer.

Season generously with pepper and salt.

Place it into the oven, then roast for at least 1 hour and 15 minutes or until golden brown and tender.

Remove from the oven and let it cool for at least 15 minutes before serving.

Nutrition:

Calories 278

Total Fat 5g,

Total Carbs 57g

Net Carbs 47g

Protein 6g

Fiber 10g

Sodium 124mg

Stir-Fried Brussels Sprouts and Carrots

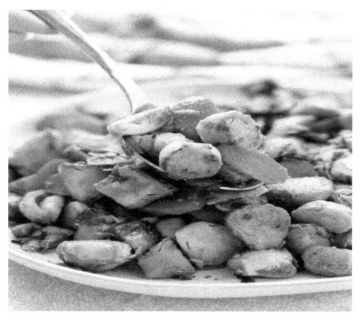

Preparation Time: 10 minutes

Cooking Time: 15 minutes

Servings: 6

Ingredients:

1 tbsp cider vinegar

1/3 cup water

1 lb. Brussels sprouts halved lengthwise

1 lb. carrots cut diagonally into ½-inch thick lengths

3 tbsp. olive oil, divided

2 tbsp. chopped shallot

½ tsp pepper

189

¾ tsp salt

Directions:

On medium-high fire, place a nonstick medium fry pan and heat 2 tbsp oil.

Ass shallots and cook until softened, around one to two minutes while occasionally stirring.

Add pepper salt, Brussels sprouts, and carrots. Stir fry until vegetables start to brown on the edges, around 3 to 4 minutes.

Add water, cook, and cover.

After 5 to 8 minutes, or when veggies are already soft, add remaining butter.

If needed, season with more pepper and salt to taste.

Turn off fire, transfer to a platter, serve and enjoy.

Nutrition:

Calories 98

 Total Fat 4g

Total Carbs 14g

Net Carbs 9g

Protein 3g

Sugar: 5g

Fiber 5g

Curried Veggies and Poached Eggs

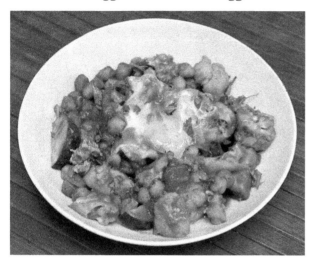

Preparation Time: 10 minutes

Cooking Time: 50 minutes

Servings: 4

Ingredients:

4 large eggs

½ tsp white vinegar

1/8 tsp crushed red pepper – optional

1 cup water

1 14-oz can chickpeas, drained

2 medium zucchinis, diced

½ lb. sliced button mushrooms

1 tbsp. yellow curry powder

2 cloves garlic, minced

191

1 large onion, chopped

2 tsp extra virgin olive oil

Directions:

On medium-high fire, place a large saucepan and heat oil.

Sauté onions until tender around four to five minutes.

Put the garlic and continue sautéing for another half minute.

Add curry powder, stir and cook until fragrant around one to two minutes.

Add mushrooms, mix, cover, and cook for 5 to 8 minutes or until mushrooms are tender and have released their liquid.

Add red pepper if using, water, chickpeas, and zucchini. Mix well to combine and bring to a boil.

Once boiling, reduce fire to a simmer, cover, and cook until zucchini is tender around 15 to 20 minutes of simmering.

Meanwhile, in a small pot filled with 3-inches deep water, bring to a boil on a high fire.

When boiling, lower the heat temperature to a simmer and add vinegar.

Slowly add one egg, slipping it gently into the water. Allow to simmer until egg is cooked, around 3 to 5 minutes.

Take off the egg using a slotted spoon and transfer to a plate, one plate one egg.

Repeat the process with remaining eggs.

 Once the veggies are done cooking, divide evenly into 4 servings and place one serving per plate of the egg.

Serve and enjoy.

Nutrition:

Calories 254

Total Fat 9g

Total Carbs 30g

Net Carbs 21g

Protein 16g

Sugar: 7g

Fiber 9g

Ground Beef with Cashews & Veggies

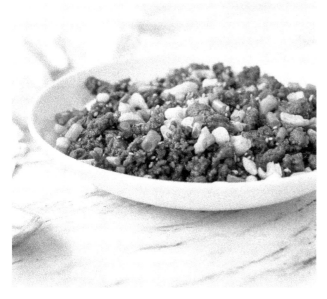

Preparation Time: 15 minutes

Cooking Time: 15 minutes

Servings: 4

Ingredients:

1½ pound lean ground beef

1 tablespoon garlic, minced

2 tablespoons fresh ginger, minced

¼ cup coconut aminos

Salt, to taste

Freshly ground black pepper, to taste

1 medium onion, sliced

1 can water chestnuts, drained and sliced

1 large green bell pepper, sliced

½ cup raw cashews, toasted

Directions:

Heat a nonstick skillet on medium-high heat.

Add beef and cook for about 6-8 minutes, breaking into pieces with all the spoon.

Add garlic, ginger, coconut aminos, salt, and black pepper and cook approximately 2 minutes.

Put the vegetables and cook approximately 5 minutes or till desired doneness.

Stir in cashews and immediately remove from heat.

Serve hot.

Nutrition:

Calories: 452

Fat: 20g

Carbohydrates: 26g

Fiber: 9g

Protein: 36g

Stuffed Trout

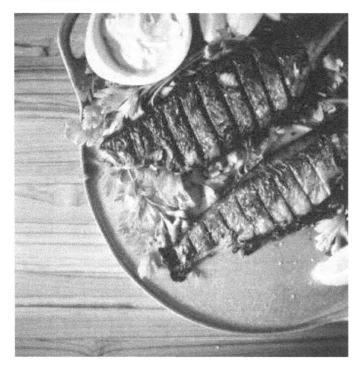

Preparation Time: 20minutes

Cooking Time: 1 hour and 15 minutes

Servings: 4

Ingredients:

1 cup chicken broth

1/2 cup quinoa

2 tablespoons omega-3-rich margarine

1 yellow onion, finely dices

1 cup (100 g) mushrooms, sliced

2 teaspoons dehydrated tarragon

Salt and pepper

1 cup cherry tomatoes, chopped

2 tablespoons lemon juice

2 tablespoons canola oil

2 whole lake trout

2 tablespoons flour

Directions:

In a pan, place the chicken broth on to simmer. Combine the quinoa, cover, and decrease the heat to low — Cook for 45 to 60 minutes.

Preheat oven to 400°F and proceed to line a baking tray with parchment paper.

To make the stuffing, melt margarine in a wide pan over medium heat. Sauté the onions and mushrooms till tender. Season by including tarragon, and salt and pepper. Combine cherry tomatoes and sauté 1 to 2 minutes further, mixing continually. Take off the heat and combine with cooked quinoa. Add in lemon juice and stir.

Spray the canola oil covering the trout. In a bowl, blend together flour, salt, and pepper. Glaze the interior and exterior of the trout with the flour batter. Stuff the trout with the stuffing blend.

Cook uncovered for 10 minutes per inch of trout.

Nutrition:

Calories: 342 kcal

Protein: 18.76 g

Fat: 19.1 g

Carbohydrates: 24.38 g

Tuna-Stuffed Tomatoes

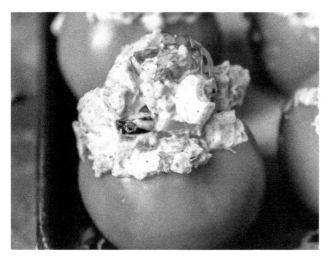

Preparation Time: 10 minutes

Cooking Time: 10 minutes

Servings: 2

Ingredients:

1 medium tomato

1 6oz. can tuna, drained and flaked

2 tbsp. mayonnaise

1 tbsp. celery, chopped

½ tsp. Dijon mustard

¼ tsp. seasoning salt

Shredded mild cheddar cheese, to garnish

Directions:

197

Preheat oven to 375°. Wash tomato and cut in half from the stem. Using a tsp., scoop out tomato pulp and any seeds until you have two ½" shells remaining.

In a small mixing bowl, combine tuna, mayonnaise, celery, mustard, and seasoning salt. Stir until well blended.

Scoop an equal amount of tuna mixture into each ½ tomato shell. Place on a baking sheet and sprinkle shredded cheddar cheese over the top of each tuna-stuffed tomato shell. Bake for 7 to 8 minutes or until cheese is melted and golden-brown in color.

Serve immediately. Any remaining mixture can be safely stored, covered, in the fridge for up to 72 hours.

Nutrition:

Calories: 175 kcal

Protein: 21.24 g

Fat: 8.79 g

Carbohydrates: 3.04 g

Seared Ahi Tuna

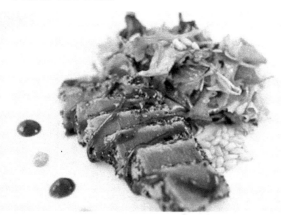

Preparation Time: 10 minutes

Cooking Time: 15 minutes

Servings: 2

Ingredients:

2 (4-ounces each) ahi tuna steaks (3/4-inch thick)

2 tbsp. dark sesame oil

2 tbsp. soy sauce

1 tbsp. of grated fresh ginger

1 clove garlic, minced

1 green onion (scallion) thinly sliced, reserve a few slices for garnish

1 tsp. lime juice

Directions:

Begin by preparing the marinade. In a small bowl, put together the sesame oil, soy sauce, fresh ginger, minced garlic, green onion, and lime juice. Mix well.

Place tuna steaks into a sealable Ziploc freezer bag and pour marinade over the top of the tuna. Seal bag and shake or massage with hands to coat tuna steaks well with marinade. Bring the bag in a bowl, in case of breaks, and place tuna in the refrigerator to marinate for at least 10 minutes.

Place a large non-stick skillet over medium-high to high heat. Let the pan heat for 2 minutes, when hot, remove tuna steaks from the marinade and lay them in the pan to sear for 1-1½ minutes on each side.

Remove tuna steaks from pan and cut into ¼-inch thick slices. Garnish with a sprinkle of sliced green onion. Serve immediately.

Nutrition:

Calories: 213 kcal

Protein: 4.5 g

Fat: 19.55 g

Carbohydrates: 5.2 g

Bavette with Seafood

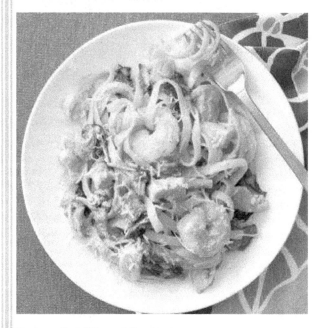

Preparation Time: 10 minutes

Cooking Time: 10 minutes

Servings: 4

Ingredients:

Braised olive oil

200g clean medium shrimp

200g of clean octopus

200g mussel without shell

200g of clean squid cut into rings

Salt to taste

Black pepper to taste

1 clove minced garlic

400g peeled tomatoes

2 tablespoons coarse salt

350g of Bavette Barilla

Chopped cilantro to taste

½ Lemon Juice

Directions:

In olive oil sauté the shrimp, the octopus, the mussel and the squid separately. Season with salt and black pepper.

In the same pan, sauté the garlic.

Add the peeled tomatoes, mix well — Cook for 2 minutes.

In a pan of boiling water, arrange 2 tablespoons of coarse salt and cook Bavette Barilla.

Remove Bavette Barilla 2 minutes before the time indicated on the package. Reserve the pasta cooking water if necessary.

Return the seafood to the sauce.

Arrange 1 scoop of the cooking water in the seafood sauce and add the drained pasta. Cook for another 2 minutes.

Finish with cilantro and lemon juice.

Serve immediately.

Nutrition:

Calories: 526 kcal

Protein: 40.59 g

Fat: 24 g

Carbohydrates: 38.02 g

Shrimp and Beets

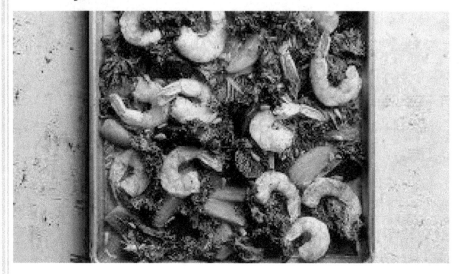

Preparation Time: 10 minutes

Cooking Time: 10 minutes

Servings: 4

Ingredients:

1 pound shrimp, peeled and deveined

2 tablespoons avocado oil

2 spring onions, chopped

2 garlic cloves, minced

1 beet, peeled and cubed

1 tablespoon lemon juice

Pinch of sea salt

Pinch of black pepper

1 teaspoon coconut aminos

Directions:

Warm a pan with the oil on medium-high heat, add the spring onions and the garlic and sauté for 2 minutes.

Add the shrimp and the other ingredients, toss, cook the mix for 8 minutes, divide into bowls and serve.

Nutrition:

Calories 281

 Fat 6g

Fiber 7g

Carbs 11g

Protein 8 g

Shrimp and Corn

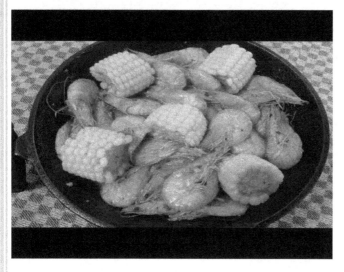

Preparation Time: 5 minutes

Cooking Time: 10 minutes

Servings: 4

Ingredients:

1 pound shrimp, peeled and deveined

2 garlic cloves, minced

1 cup corn

½ cup veggie stock

1 bunch parsley, chopped

Juice of 1 lime

2 tablespoons olive oil

204

Pinch of sea salt

Pinch of black pepper

Directions:

Warm a pan with the oil on medium-high heat, then put the garlic and the corn and sauté for 2 minutes.

Add the shrimp and the other ingredients, toss, cook everything for 8 minutes more, divide between plates and serve.

Nutrition:

Calories: 343 kcal

Protein: 29.12 g

Fat: 10.97 g

Carbohydrates: 34.25 g

Chili Shrimp and Pineapple

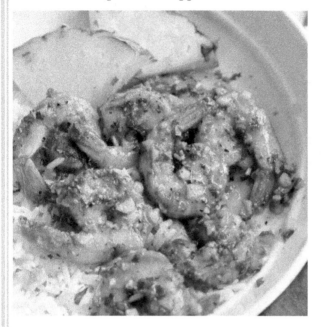

Preparation Time: 10 minutes

Cooking Time: 10 minutes

Servings: 4

Ingredients:

1 pound shrimp, peeled and deveined

2 tablespoons chili paste

Pinch of sea salt

Pinch of black pepper

1 tablespoon olive oil

1 cup pineapple, peeled and cubed

½ teaspoon ginger, grated

2 teaspoons almonds, chopped

2 tablespoons cilantro, chopped

Directions:

Warm a pan with the oil on medium-high heat, add the ginger and the chili paste, stir and cook for 2 minutes.

Add the shrimp and the other ingredients, toss, cook the mix for 8 minutes more, divide into bowls, and serve.

Nutrition:

Calories 261

Fat 4g

Fiber 7g

Carbs 15g

Protein 8g

Curry Tilapia and Beans

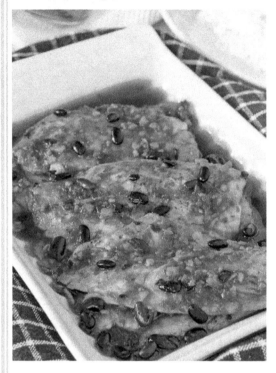

Preparation Time: 5 minutes

Cooking Time: 20 minutes

Servings: 4

Ingredients:

1 tablespoon olive oil

2 tablespoons green curry paste

4 tilapia fillets, boneless

208

Juice of ½ lime

1 cup canned red kidney beans, drained

1 tablespoon parsley, chopped

Directions:

Warm a pan with the oil on medium heat, put the fish, and cook for at least 5 minutes on each side.

Put the rest of the ingredients, toss gently, cook over medium heat for 10 minutes more, divide between plates and serve.

Nutrition:

Calories 271

Fat 4 g

Fiber 6g

Carbs 14g

Protein 7g

Balsamic Scallops

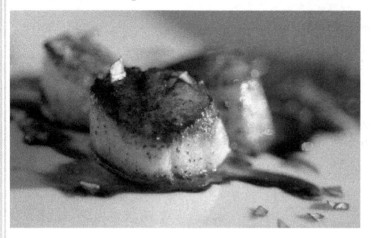

Preparation Time: 5 minutes

Cooking Time: 10 minutes

Servings: 4

Ingredients:

1 pound sea scallops

4 scallions, chopped

2 tablespoons olive oil

1 tablespoon balsamic vinegar

1 tablespoon cilantro, chopped

A pinch of salt and black pepper

Directions:

Warm a pan with the oil on medium-high heat, add the scallops, the scallions, and the other ingredients, toss, cook for 10 minutes, divide into bowls and serve.

Nutrition:

Calories 300

Fat 4g

Fiber 4g

Carbs 14g

Protein 17g

Desserts

Chocolate Chip Quinoa Granola Bars

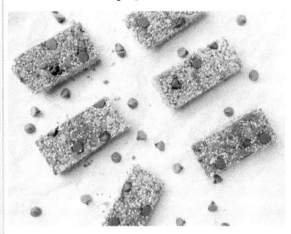

Preparation Time: 5 minutes

Cooking Time: 10 minutes

Servings: 16

Ingredients:

½ cup of chia seeds

½ cup walnuts, chopped

1 cup buckwheat

1 cup uncooked quinoa

2/3 cup dairy-free margarine

½ cup flax seed

1 teaspoon of cinnamon

½ cup of honey

½ cup of chocolate chips

1 teaspoon of vanilla

¼ teaspoon salt

Directions:

Preheat your oven to 350 degrees F.

Spread the walnuts, quinoa, wheat, flax, and chia on your baking sheet.

Bake for 10 minutes.

Line your baking dish with plastic wrap. Apply cooking spray. Keep aside.

Melt the margarine and honey in a saucepot.

Whisk together the vanilla, salt, and cinnamon into the margarine mix.

Keep the wheat mix and quinoa in a bowl. Pour the margarine sauce into it.

Stir the mixture. Coat well. Allow it to cool. Stir in the chocolate chips.

Spread your mixture into the baking dish. Press firmly into the pan.

Plastic wrap. Refrigerator overnight.

Slice into bars and serve.

Nutrition:

Calories 408

Carbohydrates 31g

Fat 28g

Protein 8g

Sugar 14g

Fiber 6g

Sodium 87mg

Strawberry Granita

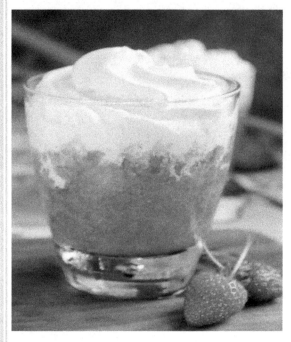

Preparation Time: 10 minutes

Cooking Time: 10 minutes

Servings: 8

Ingredients:

2 lb. strawberries, halved & hulled

1 cup of water

Agave to taste

¼ teaspoon balsamic vinegar

½ teaspoon lemon juice

Just a small pinch of salt

Directions:

Rinse the strawberries in water.

Keep in a blender. Add water, agave, balsamic vinegar, salt, and lemon juice.

Pulse many times so that the mixture moves. Blend to make it smooth.

Pour into a baking dish. The puree should be 3/8 inch deep only.

Refrigerate the dish uncovered till the edges start to freeze. The center should be slushy.

Stir crystals from the edges lightly into the center. Mix thoroughly.

Chill till the granite is almost completely frozen.

Scrape loose the crystals like before and mix.

Refrigerate again. Use a fork to stir 3-4 times till the granite has become light.

Nutrition:

Calories 72

Carbohydrates 17g

Fat 0g

Sugar 14g

Fiber 2g

Protein 1g

Apple Fritters

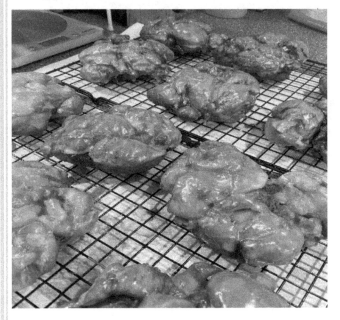

Preparation Time: 15 minutes

Cooking Time: 10 minutes

Servings: 4

Ingredients:

1 apple, cored, peeled, and chopped

1 cup all-purpose flour

1 egg

½ cup cashew milk

1-1/2 teaspoons of baking powder

2 tablespoons of stevia sugar

Directions:

216

Preheat your air fryer to 175 degrees C or 350 degrees F.

Keep parchment paper at the bottom of your fryer.

Apply cooking spray.

Mix together ¼ cup sugar, flour, baking powder, egg, milk, and salt in a bowl. Combine well by stirring.

Sprinkle 2 tablespoons of sugar on the apples. Coat well.

Combine the apples into your flour mixture.

Use a cookie scoop and drop the fritters with it to the air fryer basket's bottom.

Now air fry for 5 minutes.

Flip the fritters once and fry for another 3 minutes. They should be golden.

Nutrition:

Calories 307

Carbohydrates 65g

Total Fat 3g

Protein 5g

Sugar 39g

Fiber 2g

Sodium 248mg

Roasted Bananas

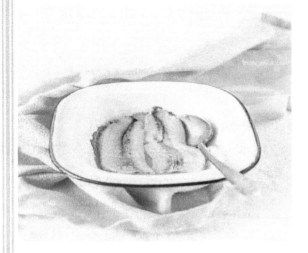

Preparation Time: 2 minutes

Cooking Time: 7 minutes

Servings: 1

Ingredients:

1 banana, sliced into diagonal pieces

Avocado oil cooking spray

Directions:

Take parchment paper and line the air fryer basket with it.

Preheat your air fryer to 190 degrees C or 375 degrees F.

Keep your slices of banana in the basket. They should not touch.

Apply avocado oil to mist the slices of banana.

Cook for 5 minutes.

Take out the basket. Flip the slices carefully.

Cook for 2 more minutes. The slices of banana should be caramelized and brown. Take them out from the basket.

Nutrition:

Calories 121

Carbohydrates 27g

Total Fat 1g

Protein 1g

Sugar 14g

Fiber 3g

Sodium 1mg

Berry-Banana Yogurt

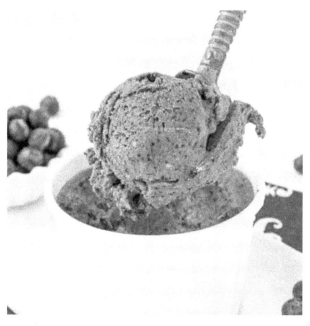

Preparation Time: 10 minutes

Cooking Time: 0 minute

Servings: 1

Ingredients:

½ banana, frozen fresh

1 container 5.3ounes Greek yogurt, non-fat

¼ cup quick-cooking oats

½ cup blueberries, fresh and frozen

1 cup almond milk

¼ cup collard greens, chopped

5-6 ice cubes

Directions:

Take microwave-safe cup and add 1 cup almond milk and ¼ cup oats

Place the cups into your microwave on high for 2.5 minutes

When oats are cooked and 2 ice cubes to cool

Mix them well

Add all ingredients in your blender

Blend it until it gets a smooth and creamy mixture

Serve chilled and enjoy!

Nutrition:

Calories: 379

Fat: 10g

Carbohydrates: 63g

Protein: 13g

Avocado Chocolate Mousse

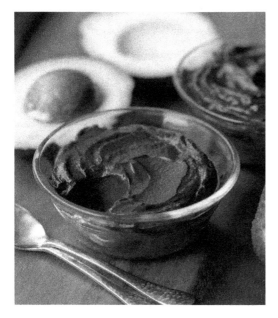

Preparation Time: 10 minutes

Cooking Time: 0 minute

Servings: 9

Ingredients:

3 ripe avocado, pitted and flesh scooped out

6 ounces plain Greek yogurt

1/8 cup almond milk, unsweetened

¼ cup espresso beans, ground

¼ cup of cocoa powder

½ teaspoon salt

2 tablespoons raw honey

221

1 bar dark chocolate

1 teaspoon vanilla extract

Directions:

Place all ingredients in your food processor

Pulse until smooth

Serve chilled and enjoy!

Nutrition:

Calories: 208

Fat: 4g

Carbohydrates: 17g

Protein: 5g

Chocolate Cherry Chia Pudding

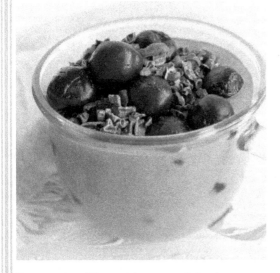

Preparation Time: 4 hours and 5 minutes

Cooking Time: 0 minutes

Servings: 4

Ingredients:

1 ½ cup Any non-dairy milk like coconut or almond milk

3 tbsp. Raw cacao powder

½ cup Sliced pitted cherries

¼ cup Chia seeds You can also use chia seed powder.

3 tbsp. Maple syrup or honey

Additional toppings:

Raw cacao nibs

Extra cherries

Dark chocolate shavings (Preferably 70% dark chocolate or more)

Directions:

Use a mason jar or a bowl. If you're using a bowl, just pour in the milk, maple syrup, chia seeds or powder, and raw cacao. Stir thoroughly and place in the refrigerator for 4 hours or more.

If you decide to use a mason jar, just pour in the same ingredients, screw the lid on and shake vigorously!

Serve in separate dishes and top with any or all of the toppings I listed above.

Enjoy!

Nutrition:

Calories: 811 kcal

Protein: 2.38 g

Fat: 83.36 g

Carbohydrates: 16.88 g

Strawberry Orange Sorbet

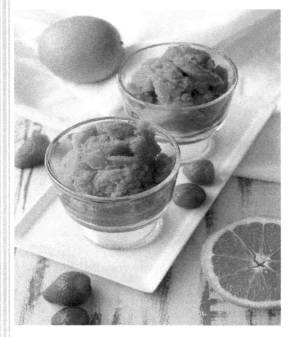

Preparation Time: 5 minutes

Cooking Time: 0 minutes

Servings: 3

Ingredients:

1 cup Orange juice or coconut water

1 pound Frozen strawberries

Direction:

Pour strawberries in a blender and pulse until all you have left are flakes. 2 minutes tops.

Now add the coconut water or orange juice and pulse until you get a nice and smooth puree. Have a spatula handy because you might need to scrape some of the puree off the walls of the blender sometimes.

Serve as soon as you're done or put in the freezer for 45 minutes for a sorbet feel.

Also, you can pour the smoothie into popsicle molds and freeze for hours or even overnight.

Enjoy!

Nutrition:

Calories: 118 kcal

Protein: 2.88 g

Fat: 2.19 g

Carbohydrates: 23.25 g

Mediterranean Rolled Baklava With Walnuts

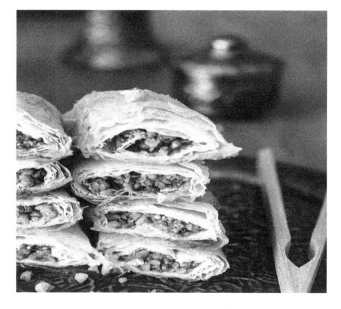

Preparation Time: 20 minutes

Cooking Time: 40 minutes

Servings: 12

Ingredients:

2 cups Walnuts

1 Lemon zest

1 cup Cream of wheat or plain breadcrumbs

8 sheets Thawed phyllo dough

3 tbsp. Sugar

1/3 cup Milk

3 sticks Melted Unsalted butter

Syrup:

1 medium Lemon

3 cups Granulated sugar

3 cups Water

Directions:

Mix 3 cups of sugar, 3 cups of water and lemon slices in a pan and leave to boil

Lower the heat, then let it simmer until the sugar completely dissolves. It should take 15 minutes. You should have a nice smooth syrup now. Now leave it to cool for a bit.

Chop the walnuts in a blender into bits using short pulses.

Pour the walnuts in a bowl along with the cream of wheat, lemon zest and 4 tablespoons of sugar.

Stir in milk and set aside.

226

Now, preheat your oven to 375°F.

Spread out the phyllo dough and fit it into a baking pan. Trim off the edges that don't fit with scissors. Cover the remaining phyllo sheets while you work so they don't dry out.

Place a sheet on a clean flat surface and glaze with melted butter. Do this for all the sheets until it's finished.

Arrange the walnut mixture on one side of the sheets and roll them up like you're trying to make a sausage. Do this for all the sheets and walnuts.

Arrange the walnut rolls on an ungreased baking pan and glaze with the leftover butter.

Bake for about 45 minutes. It's ready when it looks golden.

Turn off the oven then pull out the baking pan. Drizzle syrup over the baklava, making sure the syrup gets everywhere.

Bring back the baking pan into the oven then leave to sit for 5 minutes.

Take off from the oven and leave it to cool for a few hours. Slice the rolls into tiny bits and serve.

Nutrition:

Calories: 488 kcal

Protein: 4.49 g

Fat: 36.89 g

Carbohydrates: 38.21 g

Mint Chocolate Chip Ice-cream

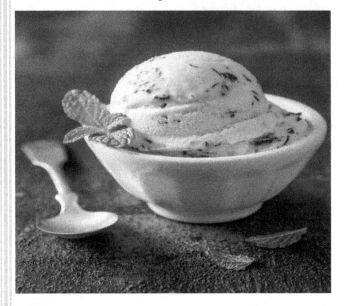

Preparation Time: 5 minutes

Cooking Time: 0 minutes

Servings: 2

Ingredients:

2 Frozen overripe bananas

Pinch Spirulina or any natural food coloring, optional.

3 tbsp. Chocolate chips or sugar-free chocolate chips

1/8 tsp. Pure peppermint extract

½ cup Raw cashews or coconut cream, optional.

Pinch Salt

Directions:

Mint or imitation peppermint won't be a substitute for this. Use pure peppermint extract and pour it all at once because a drop is more potent than you realize, so add slowly.

Peel and cut the bananas first. Place the slices in a Ziplock bag then freeze.

For the ice cream, put all the ingredients in a blender and pulse. You can skip the chocolate chips and just add them after blending. It'll turn out delicious either way.

Serve as soon as it's ready or freeze until it's firm enough, then serve!

Nutrition:

Calories: 250 kcal

Protein: 6.13 g

Fat: 24.37 g

Carbohydrates: 7.72 g

Flourless Sweet Potato Brownies

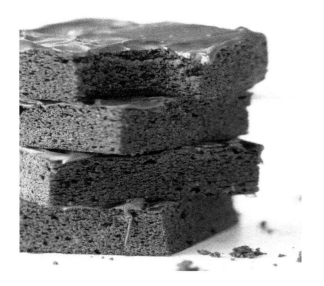

Preparation Time: 10 minutes

Cooking Time: 30 minutes

Servings: 9

Ingredients:

½ cup Cooked sweet potato

2 tsp. Vanilla extract

½ cup Almond butter

6 tbsp. Honey

½ tsp. Baking soda

1 large Whole egg

¼ cup Unsweetened Cocoa powder

3 tbsp. Dairy-free chocolate chips, optional.

Directions:

Prep your oven by preheating to 350°F.

Line a baking pan with parchment paper leaving a few extra inches on the sides to make it easier to discard or remove

Blend all the ingredients, excluding the chocolate chips until you get a very smooth and soft batter.

Transfer the creamy batter to your prepared baking pan and use a spatula to spread it around, so it looks almost even.

Slide it in the oven, then bake for 30 minutes or until a knife inserted into the pan comes out clean.

Take off from the oven and leave to cool in the pan for 15 minutes before putting it up on a wire rack.

If you decide to use the chocolate chip topping, put the chips in a microwave-safe dish and heat until it completely melts. Take off from the microwave and drizzle over the brownies.

Serve or store!

Nutrition:

Calories: 171 kcal

Protein: 5.17 g

Fat: 9.28 g

Carbohydrates: 20.01 g

Paleo Raspberry Cream Pie

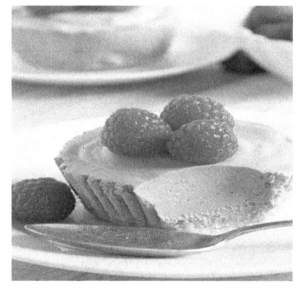

Preparation Time: 20 minutes

Cooking Time: 0 minutes

Servings: 12

Ingredients:

231

For the crust:

1 ½ tbsp. Maple syrup

Pinch Salt

½ cup Unsweetened shredded coconut

1 tsp. Vanilla extract

1 cup Roasted or salted cashews

Raspberry filling:

¾ cup Unrefined coconut oil

1 ½ cup Roasted or salted cashews

½ cup & 1 tbsp. Maple syrup

¼ cup & 2 tsp. Fresh lemon juice

¼ cup Coconut cream from the top solid part of a can of coconut milk that has been refrigerated overnight

2 tsp. Vanilla extract

3 cups Fresh raspberries

Pinch Salt

Directions:

Prepare 12 muffin pans, line them with muffin liners, and set them aside.

Make the crust. Set a pan over medium heat and the coconut and stir until it's completely toasted. Stay by the pan because coconuts tend to burn very easily.

Transfer the toasted coconuts to a bowl and leave to cool for 5 minutes or so. Honestly, this toasting step isn't particularly necessary, but I feel it adds amazing flavor to the crust.

To make the crust, put all the ingredients in a blender and pulse at the lowest speed until the mix gets all clumpy. Also, don't pulse for too long, or you might end up with a paste. To know if it's ready, put a bit of the mixture on your fingers and pinch. If it gets clumpy, you're on track, if not, add a little water and pulse at the lowest speed for further minutes.

Scoop the mix into the lined tins using your fingers to pack the mix tightly inside the pan.

Put the pans to refrigerate while you get to make the filling.

In a tiny pot set over low heat, stir in all the ingredients until the oil and coconut cream melts completely. Clean the blender using a paper towel and pour in the filling.

Pulse at high-speed for like 60 seconds or until it's completely smooth. The only clumps we can forgive are the raspberry seeds.

Drizzle a quarter of the filling over the top of each crust. There should be extra filling; you can store and use that in another dish.

Place the coated muffins in the fridge to cool. This will take a few hours, like 6 hours, so if you don't have time for that, put it in the freezer.

To serve, leave them to defrost for 80 minutes or until obviously creamy.

Nutrition:

Calories: 565 kcal

Protein: 7.74 g

Fat: 43.72 g

Carbohydrates: 42.72 g

Caramelized Pears

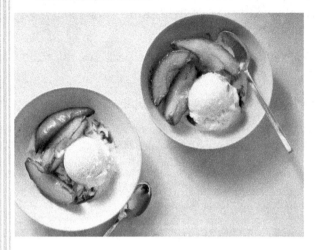

Preparation Time: 20 minutes

Cooking Time: 5 minutes

Servings: 5

Ingredients:

1 Teaspoon Cinnamon

2 Tablespoon Honey, Raw

1 Tablespoon Coconut Oil

4 Pears, Peeled, Cored & Quartered

2 Cups Yogurt, Plain

¼ Cup Toasted Pecans, Chopped

1/8 Teaspoon Sea Salt

Directions:

Get out a large skillet, and then heat the oil over medium-high heat.

Add in your honey, cinnamon, pears, and salt. Cover, and allow it to cook for four to five minutes. Stir occasionally, and your fruit should be tender.

Uncover it, and allow the sauce to simmer until it thickens. This will take several minutes.

Soon your yogurt into four dessert bowls. Top with pears and pecans before serving.

Nutrition:

Calories: 290

Protein: 12 g

Fat: 11 g

Carbs: 41 g

Anti-Inflammatory Apricot Squares

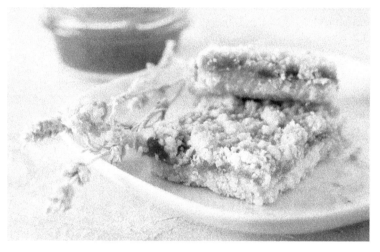

Preparation Time: 20 minutes

Cooking Time: 0 minute

Servings: 8

Ingredients:

1 cup shredded coconut, dried

1 teaspoon vanilla extract

1 cup apricot, dried

1 cup macadamia nuts, chopped

1 cup apricot, chopped

1/3 cup turmeric powder

Directions:

Place all ingredients in your food processor

Pulse until smooth

Place the mixture into a square pan and press evenly

Serve chilled and enjoy!

Nutrition:

Calories: 201

Fat: 15g

Carbohydrates: 17g

Protein: 3g

Raw Black Forest Brownies

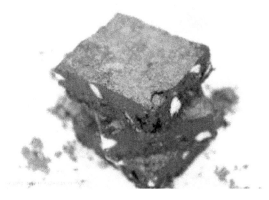

Preparation Time: 2 hours and 10 minutes

Cooking Time: 0 minute

Servings: 6

Ingredients:

1 and ½ cups cherries, pitted, dried and chopped

1 cup raw cacao powder

½ cup dates pitted

2 cups walnuts, chopped

½ cup almonds, chopped

¼ teaspoon salt

Directions:

Place all ingredients in your food processor

Pulse until small crumbs are formed

Press the brownie batter in a pan

Freeze for two hours

Slice before serving and enjoy!

Nutrition:

Calories: 294

Fat: 18g

Carbohydrates: 33g

Protein: 7g

Berry Parfait

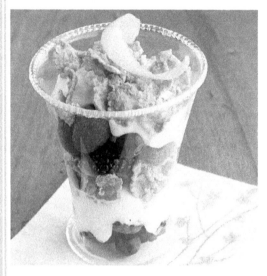

Preparation Time: 10 minutes

Cooking time: 10 minutes

Servings: 5

Ingredients:

7oz / 200g almond butter

3.5oz / 100g Greek yogurt

14oz / 400g mixed berries

2 tsp honey

7oz / 200g mixed nuts

Directions:

Mix the Greek yogurt, butter, and honey until its smooth.

Add a layer of berries and a layer of the mixture in a glass until it's full.

Serve immediately with sprinkled nuts.

Nutrition:

Calories: 250

Carbohydrates: 17 g

Protein: 7.2 g

Fat: 19.4 g

Sugar: 42.3 g

Fiber: 6.6 g

Sodium: 21 mg

Sherbet Pineapple

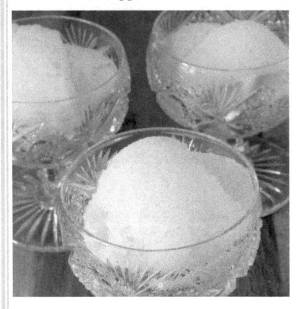

Preparation Time: 20 minutes

Cooking Time: 0 minutes

Servings: 4

Ingredients:

1 can of 8-ounce pineapple chunks

1/3 cup of orange marmalade

¼ teaspoon of ground ginger

¼ teaspoon of vanilla extract

1 can of 11-ounce orange sections

2 cups of pineapple, lemon or lime sherbet

Directions:

Drain the pineapple, ensure you reserve the juice.

Take a medium-sized bowl and add pineapple juice, ginger, vanilla and marmalade to the bowl

Add pineapple chunks, drained mandarin oranges as well

Toss well and coat everything

Free them for 15 minutes and allow them to chill

Spoon the sherbet into 4 chilled stemmed sherbet dishes

Top each of them with fruit mixture

Enjoy!

Nutrition:

Calories: 267 Cal

Fat: 1 g

Carbohydrates: 65 g

Protein: 2 g

Easy Peach Cobbler

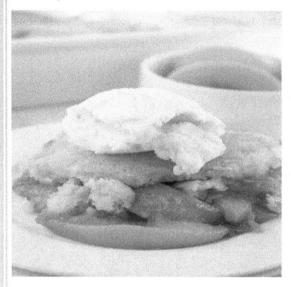

Preparation Time: 5 minutes

Cooking Time: 20 minutes

Servings: 6

Ingredients:

5 organic peaches, pitted and chopped

¼ cup coconut palm sugar, divided

½ teaspoon cinnamon

¾ cup chopped pecans

½ cup gluten-free oats

¼ cup ground flaxseeds

¼ brown rice flour

¼ cup extra virgin olive oil

Directions:

Preheat the oven to 3500F.

Grease the bottom of 6 ramekins.

In a bowl, mix the peaches, ½ of the coconut sugar, cinnamon, and pecans.

Distribute the peach mixture into the ramekins.

In the same bowl, mix the oats, flaxseed, rice flour, and oil. Add in the remaining coconut sugar. Mix until a crumbly texture is formed.

Top the mixture over the peaches.

Place for 20 minutes.

Nutrition:

Calories 26

 Fat: 11g

 Carbohydrates: 28g

Protein: 10g

Sugar: 12g

Fiber: 6g

Drinks

Blueberry Matcha Smoothie

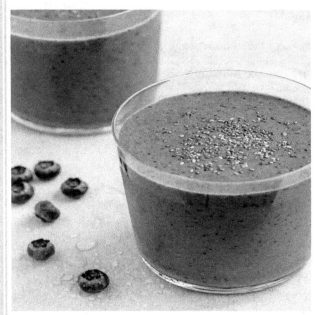

Preparation Time: 5 minutes

Cooking Time: 0 minutes

Servings: 2

Ingredients:

2 Cups Blueberries, Frozen

2 Cups Almond Milk

1 Banana

2 Tablespoons Protein Powder, Optional

¼ Teaspoon Ground Cinnamon

1 Tablespoon Chia Seeds

1 Tablespoon Matcha Powder

¼ Teaspoon Ground Ginger

A Pinch Sea Salt

Directions:

Blend everything until smooth.

Nutrition:

Calories: 208

Protein: 8.7 g

Fat: 5.7 g

Carbs: 31 g

Pumpkin Pie Smoothie

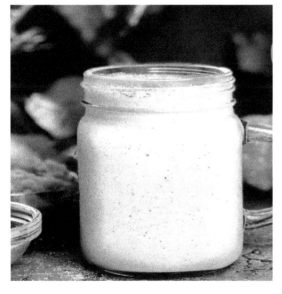

Preparation Time: 5 minutes

Cooking Time: 0 minutes

Servings: 2

Ingredients:

1 Banana

½ Cup Pumpkin, Canned & Unsweetened

2-3 Ice Cubes

1 Cup Almond Milk

2 Tablespoons Almond Butter, Heaping

1 Teaspoon Ground Nutmeg

1 Teaspoon Ground Cinnamon

1 Teaspoon Vanilla Extract Pure

1 Teaspoon Maple Syrup, Pure

Directions:

Blend everything together until smooth.

Nutrition:

Calories: 235

Protein: 5.6 g

Fat: 11 g

Carbs: 27.8 g

Fig Smoothie

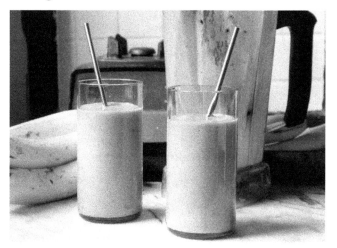

Preparation Time: 5 minutes

Cooking Time: 0 minutes

Servings: 2

Ingredients:

7 Figs, Halved (Fresh or Frozen)

1 Banana

1 Cup Whole Milk Yogurt, Plain

1 Cup Almond Milk

1 Teaspoon Flaxseed, Ground

1 Tablespoon Almond Butter

1 Teaspoon Honey, Raw

3-4 Ice Cubes

Directions:

Blend all together ingredients until smooth, and serve immediately.

Nutrition:

Calories: 362

Protein: 9 g

Fat: 12 g

Carbs: 60 g

Blended Coconut Milk and Banana Breakfast Smoothie

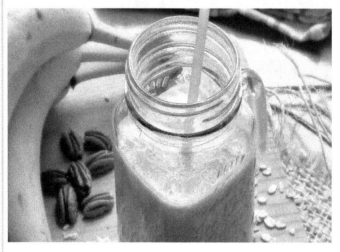

Preparation Time: 10 minutes

Cooking Time: 0 minutes

Servings: 4

Ingredients:

4 ripe medium-sized bananas

4 tbsp. flax seeds

2 cups almond milk

2 cups coconut milk

4 tsp. cinnamon

Directions:

Peel the banana and slice it into ½-inch pieces. Put all the ingredients in the blender and blend into a smoothie. Add a dash of cinnamon at the top of the smoothie before serving.

Nutrition:

Calories: 332 kcal

Protein: 12.49 g

Fat: 14.42 g

Carbohydrates: 42.46 g

Kale Smoothie

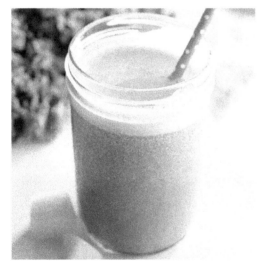

Preparation Time: 10 minutes

Cooking Time: 0 minutes

Servings: 2

Ingredients:

10 kale leaves

5 bananas, peeled and cut into chunks

2 pears, chopped

5 tbsp. almond butter

5 cups almond milk

Directions:

In your blender, mix the kale with the bananas, pears, almond butter, and almond milk.

Pulse well, divide into glasses, and serve. Enjoy!

Nutrition:

Calories: 267

Fat: 11 g

Protein: 7 g

Carbs: 15 g

Fiber: 7 g

Raspberry Smoothie

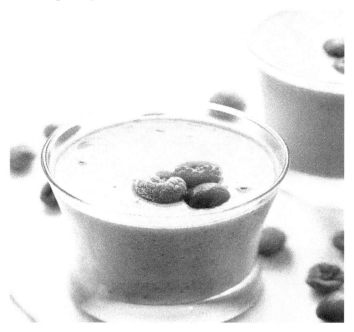

Preparation Time: 10 minutes

Cooking Time: 0 minutes

Servings: 2

Ingredients:

1 avocado, pitted and peeled

3/4 cup raspberry juice

3/4 cup orange juice

1/2 cup raspberries

Directions:

In your blender, mix the avocado with the raspberry juice, orange juice, and raspberries.

Pulse well, divide into 2 glasses, and serve. Enjoy!

Nutrition:

Calories: 125

Fat: 11 g

Protein: 3 g

Carbs: 9 g

Fiber: 7 g

Pineapple Smoothie

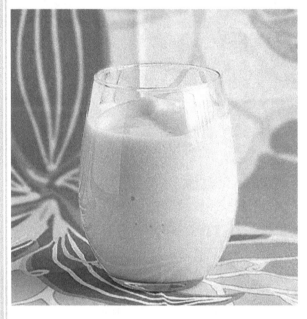

Preparation Time: 10 minutes

Cooking Time: 0 minutes

Servings: 2

Ingredients:

1 cup coconut water

1 orange, peeled and cut into quarters

1 1/2 cups pineapple chunks

1 tbsp. fresh grated ginger

1 tsp. chia seeds

1 tsp. turmeric powder

A pinch black pepper

Directions:

In your blender, mix the coconut water with the orange, pineapple, ginger, chia seeds, turmeric, and black pepper.

Pulse well, pour into a glass.

Serve for breakfast. Enjoy!

Nutrition:

Calories: 151

Fat: 2 g

Protein: 4 g

Carbs: 12 g

Fiber: 6 g

Almond Blueberry Smoothie

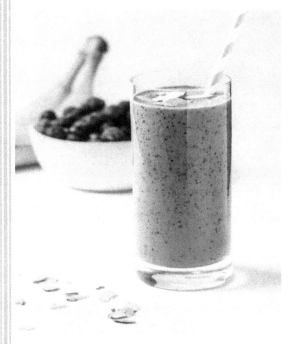

Preparation Time: 10 minutes

Cooking Time: 0 minutes

Servings: 1

Ingredients:

1 cup frozen blueberries

1 banana

1/2 cup almond milk

1 tbsp. almond butter

Water, as needed

Directions:

Add everything to a blender jug.

Cover the jug tightly.

Blend until smooth. Serve and enjoy!

Nutrition:

Calories: 211

Fat: 0.2 g

Protein: 5.6 g

Carbs: 3.4 g

Fiber: 2.3 g

Green Vanilla Smoothie

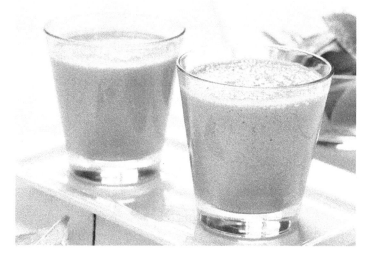

Preparation Time: 10 minutes

Cooking Time: 0 minutes

Servings: 1

Ingredients:

1 banana, cut in chunks

1 cup grapes

1 tub (6 oz.) vanilla yogurt

1/2 apple, cored and chopped

1 1/2 cups fresh spinach leaves

Directions:

Add everything to a blender jug.

Cover the jug tightly.

Blend until smooth. Serve and enjoy!

Nutrition:

Calories: 131

Fat: 0.2 g

Protein: 2.6 g

Carbs: 9.1 g

Fiber: 1.3 g

Vanilla Blueberry Smoothie

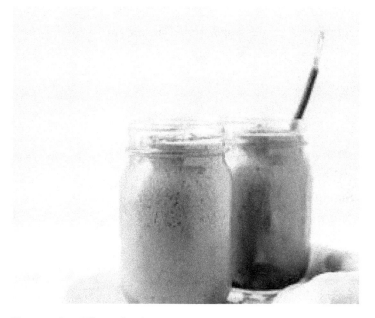

Preparation Time: 5 minutes

Cooking Time: 0 minutes

Servings: 1

Ingredients:

2 cups hemp milk

1 cup fresh blueberries

 Handful of ice/ 1 cup frozen blueberries

 1 tbsp. flaxseed oil

2 tbsp. hemp protein powder

Directions:

257

Combine milk and fresh blueberries plus ice (or frozen blueberries) in a blender.

Blend for 1 minute, transfer to a glass, and stir in flaxseed oil.

Nutrition:

Calories: 1041 kcal

Protein: 35.21 g

Fat: 41.04 g

Carbohydrates: 140.4 g

Zesty Citrus Smoothie

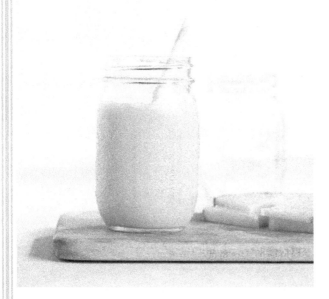

Preparation Time: 5 minutes

Cooking Time: 0 minutes

Servings: 1

Ingredients:

1 cup almond milk

half cup lemon juice

1 med orange peeled, cleaned, and sliced into sections

Handful of ice

1 tbsp. flaxseed oil

2 tsp hemp protein powder

Directions:

Combine milk, lemon juice, orange, and ice in a blender.

Blend for 1 minute, transfer to a glass, and stir in flaxseed oil.

Nutrition:

Calories: 427 kcal

Protein: 17.5 g

Fat: 28.88 g

Carbohydrates: 24.96 g

Conclusion

All throughout the world, people struggle with pain and disease. But diseases are rising at a shocking rate in many Western countries. Despite having advanced medical facilities, people are developing illnesses at a shocking rate. While there are many causes for these illnesses, studies have found that one major cause is inflammation. This inflammation can cause a person to develop arthritis, heart disease, Alzheimer's disease, and so much more. Not only that, but many people are living their day to day lives in pain, struggling to get enough sleep, and overly stressed.

This can be overwhelming to take in, but the good news is that by following the anti-inflammatory diet, you can improve your health. You can live the life you have dreamed of. Whether you hope to decrease your risk of common diseases or improve your everyday life, you can trust in knowing that science has shown the anti-inflammatory diet to be the answer.

It can be difficult to start a new lifestyle, but it doesn't have to be. By using the information in this book, trying out the recipes, and following the menu plan, you can easily practice the anti-inflammatory diet with ease. You can adjust your lifestyle without worry or stress, simply allowing yourself to enjoy a delicious meal after delicious meal. Of course, remember that the anti-inflammatory diet is not only about food. It is a lifestyle approach, meaning you should also try to implement healthy exercise, sleep, and any needed supplements as advised by your doctor. By approaching this as a lifestyle rather than a diet, you can gain the holistic benefits you desire.

CPSIA information can be obtained
at www.ICGtesting.com
Printed in the USA
BVHW092104060721
611233BV00002B/353